STOPPING
KIDNEY DISEASE
FOOD GUIDE

LEE HULL

Recipe videos, new recipes, and written instructions
for recipe videos can be downloaded here:

https://kidneyhood.org/pages/kidney-friendly-recipes

Stopping Kidney Disease Food Guide

PUBLISHED BY KIDNEYHOOD.ORG

First edition, May 2019

All rights reserved.

ISBN: 978-0-578-49362-6

Table of Contents

About the Author

Lee Hull has been a kidney patient for the past twenty-two years, the first twelve of which he spent trying to cure an incurable kidney disease. Lee went into remission ten years ago and has stayed in remission using the treatment and diet plan in this book.

Why another kidney diet or meal planning book?

It's simple. We as patients want our kidneys to last as long as possible, and we want to live longer and better lives. We want a cure, but if we can't get a cure we want to slow the kidney disease progression to a snail's pace. That's what we want and deserve.

The problem is today's kidney diets have nothing in common with our real goals.

Let us list some reasons why it's time for a change:

1. Current kidney disease diets are based on information that is 50 years old (1960s and 1970s) and not on today's latest research (2018/2019).

2. Current kidney disease diets act as if only three issues matter: potassium, phosphorus, and sodium. This concept is not true and does not stand up to even the smallest amount of scrutiny.

3. Current kidney disease diets are full of conflicting ideas that may result in more problems than they solve. For example, these diets use meat as a source of protein. The metabolism of dietary protein creates uremia, uremic toxins, acidosis, increased renal acid load, and inflammation, all of which increase the speed of kidney disease progression. Yes, we did limit sodium, potassium, and phosphorus, but at what cost? Did we gain anything by managing three conditions, but creating three or four more? In many cases, we contribute to uremic malnutrition instead of preventing it.

4. Current kidney diets do not address issues like antioxidants, acidosis, renal acid load, keto acids, polyphenols, advanced glycation end (AGE) products, inflammation, and the list goes on. Yet, all of these factors can speed or slow kidney disease progression.

The bottom line is that the current kidney diets are killing us. I am not being dramatic; keep reading and I will explain.

Current diets keep our renal acid load and protein workload the same throughout our disease progression. No recognition is made that our kidneys can no longer handle this workload. This fact speeds the progression of kidney disease over time.

I admit to being touchy on this topic after my experience as a 20+ year kidney patient. I mention this because I have spent more than two decades in the trenches and have, by almost all standards, been a very successful kidney patient. I have maintained my kidneys for over 20 years, despite having an incurable form of kidney disease.

The recipes and eating plan in this book are based on the research in *Stopping Kidney Disease*. This book is meant to be a companion book to *Stopping Kidney Disease*. Hundreds of studies and medical trials point us in the same direction over and over again. Some of these subjects have never been presented to kidney patients before like renal acid load. It's time for us to have an up to date, well researched diet and plan for slowing or maybe even stopping our disease. We need to treat every factor we can possibly treat, not just three.

I am trying to keep this book cheap and affordable so I will not be reprinting chapters from "Stopping Kidney Disease". The number of color pages increases the printing prices dramatically, so short and sweet will be the theme here.

Your education will determine your outcome and odds.

If you learn one thing from this book or other books in this series, it should be:

Educated patients live longer and better lives. Education on your disease and treatment options will likely be the greatest factor in your success or failure in dealing with this disease.

I have tried it all: drugs, diets, the best hospitals in the US, and even traveled overseas for help. I am here to tell you as a fellow patient that it is very likely that everything you know about kidney diets is wrong, or if it's "right," it is 50 years behind the times. As I said, most of our current guidelines can be traced back to the 1950s, 60s, and 70s.

An analogy of our current dietary situation might help:

> Assume you are in an accident and break ten bones, but the doctors decided 50 years ago that the maximum they can treat is three broken bones. Seven bones go untreated because that's the way they did it 50 years ago.

Traditional and other current kidney diets focus on treating just three conditions as we all know: sodium, phosphorus, and potassium. However, most of us have many more comorbid conditions made worse by traditional kidney diets. We need to try and treat, cure or manage as many conditions as possible, not just three. You would never know you need treat other conditions or have other dietary options unless you get educated.

Patient-to-Patient, the fastest and best hope for us

The reasons why I am so focused on educating patients and caregivers is time, location, apathy, and improving your odds regardless of where you live.

Change is painfully slow in all areas, but medical related changes takes decades. Nutrition research seem to be especially dominated by marketing and trendy foods, not facts for kidney patients.

It took 40 years and over 7,000 studies before smoking was declared bad for us.

It takes 12 to 20 years for a drug to make it to the marketplace.

According to the Institute of Medicine in their Yearbook of Medical Informatics, it takes 17 years for a new medical practice to be adopted.

No matter what data you review, change takes decades. The well-meaning and nice people who are advising us are woefully behind the times. It's not their fault; it's the system that we have and we have to deal with it.

I believe patient-to-patient help and education is the answer. The reason is, we will all die waiting for our caregivers to catch up with current information. I didn't have 15 or 20 years to wait for a cure or a way to slow my disease.

This is even more of a factor as most kidney patients are over 60 years of age. Waiting 20 years is not an option for us.

We are motivated to find a solution, to find something that works, and to find a way to live longer and better. We have our entire skin in the game. We are all in whether we like it or not. Those helping us don't have this kind of pressure and motivation. Our caregivers are also constrained by rules and regulations, but we patients are not. We are free to search and try alternatives our caregivers will not hear about until decades later.

Patient-to-patient education allows you to get educated today, not 20 years from now. Education needed for lots of reasons and apathy is one of them.

Apathy

If you want proof, listen to my experience in the past 45 days:

After publishing *Stopping Kidney Disease*, I was surprised by the number of emails and calls I got about caregivers (doctors, nutritionists, dietitians, even dialysis clinics) telling patients things like "It can't work or I would know about it" or "I am sorry, but whatever they are saying won't help you." I went out of my way in *Stopping Kidney Disease* to cite over 700 medical studies because I knew this would happen. Yet, hundreds or even thousands of studies are not enough to convince caregivers that it is 2019, not 1950.

> I have gotten involved in a few of these by accident. A few patients called me while at a doctors or nutritionist appointment. I was asked to talk about the diet and treatment plan after the caregivers said "No."

My response to caregivers is the same:

"I am not a doctor but the patient has an incurable disease and other treatments have failed or are not available. It takes only 90 days to find out if the plan will help them. Eating a diet to try to treat your disease and retesting your bloodwork in 90 days is not radical or extreme. It's the least risky and lowest cost option, and likely the only one they have left. Why in the world would you tell a patient "No"?

"Have you read the book and looked at the research?"

"100% of the time, the response has been something along these lines: "Oh, well when you put it that way, I see no harm in trying it" and "No, I have not looked at the book."

Think about this for a moment: We, the patient, might die 30 years prematurely and have all kinds of medical problems and wipe out our family with medical bills during these years, but in an instant with no research, no questioning, no nothing, our request is dismissed without a thought about us at all. In a 60-second conversation, a caregiver can go from "no" to "yes." Our caregivers don't think twice about the implications of a snap and very uninformed decision that could take or add years to our life.

I personally believe dialysis (while needed and lifesaving) has crippled progress in kidney disease research. We have a backup plan that will keep us alive; no other disease has this backup plan. It's not uncommon for cancer patients to try many treatments including new and experimental treatments. There is no equivalent of dialysis for other deadly diseases, so everything is on the table for them. For us, it is assumed we can just go on dialysis someday; there's no need to trying anything new or different.

As I stated, I get these kinds of emails and calls each week:

My doctor, dialysis clinic, nutritionist, or someone else told me the information in *Stopping Kidney Disease* won't work. They want me to stick with their current diet and treatment plan, so I am going to do what they say. There may be nothing wrong with this decision, but let's talk about blind acceptance a little more.

This happens every day, as only a fraction of patients contact us, but let's think about the consequences of this decision for a second. Ok, nice people are advising you and many of us blindly accept their recommendations despite not getting better or the results we want.

What if this blind acceptance takes years off your life? I lost a dear friend due to this kind of blind acceptance. What if this advice is causing you to drive 100 mph toward kidney failure and all kinds of comorbid conditions? You end up in a very bad place because of blind acceptance and trust despite hundreds of studies suggesting a different approach might help you.

I can give you two very personal stories about blind acceptance vs education. The first is the one you already know, my struggle to get help with my kidney disease. The second is about my youngest son, Lucas, and autism.

In 2011, we had just finished building our dream house in Texas. We had been living in the house for 18 months when we dropped everything and moved to Wisconsin.

Our youngest son was diagnosed with autism in April of 2012. Based on my experience with kidney disease, I started researching autism treatments and burning up the phones setting up appointments to get second opinions and advice. What we found out shocked us. The state and town had very little support infrastructure or therapy programs. In fact, at the time there were only two states in the country in which insurance covered intensive autism therapy and whose programs had a track record. Other states had some things covered and other things were not covered. It was almost impossible to figure out what would be covered and what wouldn't be covered. In addition to this chaos, strong debates existed on the best way to treat autism. No one seems to know which approach was best and no standard treatment existed. The out of pocket estimates were anywhere from $65,000 to over $85,000 per year in costs if insurance would not cover treatment.

We couldn't be sure of anything, cost or effectiveness of certain treatment theory etc...

Then, it turns out there was one open spot for a two year old 1,000 miles away and another opening could be six+ months away. My wife and I talked that night and started the move to Wisconsin the next day. 87 days later, we were living in an extended stay hotel while he started therapy in the hotel room while we looked for a house in the right school district for our kids.

Four years and eight months after the move, I got a letter stating that an opening was available back in Texas. My son is now nine and has completed over 6,800+ hours of therapy. A child who pointed to everything because he couldn't speak is now doing great in school and doing things we thought impossible a few years ago. Two weeks ago, he skied every hill at the local ski hill. Two years ago, he freaked out getting snow on any part of this body. Three years ago, he had to wear headphones at choir practice or music lessons. Today, he loves music and goes to every school event and dances for hours. He still has issues we will be working on for years to come, but the change is nothing short of remarkable. We have gone from a child not speaking to one is now very likely to have a pretty normal life.

The " expert" advice in Texas was to get on the waiting list for therapy and to keep our expectations very low for our son. If we had followed this advice, we would have missed four and a half years of early intervention therapy totaling around 4,000+ hours.

Our doctors, some family, and friends thought we were losing our mind for such a sudden move after building a house we thought we would be in for decades. Everyone told us we were overreacting and to not make a rash decision. The word "hysterical" was used more than once. The most common advice was " wait a few years and see what happens first."

For the record, "wait and see" is the shittiest advice in the world when it comes to helping a child. It's never wrong to do everything possible to help a child as early as possible. We had no guarantees of success or improvement. We also knew nothing bad would come from intensive therapy. Our perspective was this was a very low risk bet. Worst case, nothing changed and we moved for nothing. The best case scenario would be life changing for our son. What looked like hysteria to family and friends was a very informed decision on our part.

Why I am telling you this story? Kidney disease is similar in many ways. Your doctor will likely recommend a wait and see approach. No standard treatment exists for incurable kidney disease. You have no guarantee of success either. In addition to these facts, where you live may dramatically affect your treatment options and the advice you get just like my son. If we had lived in a different city, state or country the "expert's" advice would have been very different. This also means your outcome will be greatly affected by the "experts" in your area.

Our decision to move was based on our crash course in autism, autism treatment theories, and insurance coverage. Education and lack of other options drove our decision to pick up and move without any guarantees.

The situation is no different for kidney patients. If you don't get educated, you won't have access to all treatment options, and even if you get educated there are no guarantees. I recently was questioned by a nephrologist on the concept that kidney disease advice and outcomes will vary greatly by location. He felt advice was very standardized. I had no proof at the time. I had my personal experience and the experiences of hundreds of other patients, but no concrete facts until now.

The following is from the Center for Disease Control (CDC) 2017 study on kidney disease mortality by state. I then matched up a few countries and states based on a similar study by the World Health Organization.

Location	Kidney Disease Death per 100,000 in population	Country Equivalent
Mississippi	21.7	Nepal
Louisiana	20.6	Mexico
Arkansas	19.7	Argentina
Missouri	19.6	Chad
Kentucky	19.4	Qatar
Georgia	18.6	
Indiana	18.5	
West Virginia	17.1	
North Carolina	17.0	
Virginia	16.9	
Illinois	16.8	
Alabama	16.5	
Delaware	16.1	
Texas	16.0	
Pennsylvania	15.9	
South Carolina	15.5	
Utah	15.3	
Kansas	15.0	
Ohio	15.0	
Michigan	14.7	

Location	Kidney Disease Death per 100,000 in population	Country Equivalent
Tennessee	14.4	
New Jersey	13.9	
Massachusetts	13.4	
Maine	13.0	
New Mexico (25th)	12.9	Iran
North Dakota	12.9	
Wisconsin	12.5	
Maryland	11.9	
Rhode Island	11.6	
Connecticut	11.2	
Hawaii	10.7	
Oklahoma	10.2	
Florida	10.1	
Alaska	9.9	
Nebraska	9.5	
Wyoming	9.5	
New Hampshire	9.4	
Montana	9.2	
New York	9.1	
Idaho	9.0	
Nevada	9.0	
California	8.9	
Colorado	8.9	
Iowa	8.8	
Minnesota	7.7	
Oregon	7.3	Zambia
South Dakota	6.8	Portugal
Arizona	6.2	Kenya
Washington	5.2	Norway
Vermont	3.3	Finland

A few things stick out:

You are 700% more likely to die from kidney disease in Mississippi than Vermont.

Many states (and the U.S.) as a whole are third-world countries in terms of kidney outcomes.

While I can't explain all of the reasons for these numbers, I can tell you how to solve the problem: Education of the patient. An educated patient can turn a third-world country into first-class medical care if they understand their treatment options and are willing to invest some time in getting educated. We are watching this happen in real time. Stopping Kidney Disease and Albutrix are being ordered from Singapore to South Africa. The availability of treatment and access to medical care is different in each country. However, an educated patient can level the field and get access to options that uneducated patients may not be aware of. It doesn't cost much to get educated either.

I will say it again, patient education is the fastest route to leveling the playing field and getting every kidney patient access to treatment options that may extend the life of your kidneys and your life as well. Regardless of where you live, your net worth, or formal education you can become an expert on what works for you and try every treatment option you can find if you are educated on your disease and your kidneys.

Math and GFR

As a part of your education, you need to understand the mathematics of delaying disease progression. Every small difference matters over the years and decades. Some may question this validity of delaying or slowing disease progression. If they do, they have not taken the time to get educated.

Assume your GFR is 40 today. What happens to the lifespan of your kidneys with different disease progression rates? We will say a GFR of 10 is dialysis or kidney failure. You might say you have 30 GFR points to work with. How far can an educated patient get on 30 GFR points? We are not counting the current year or the year your GFR hits 10. We are only counting the years of decline until we hit a GFR of 10.

Average GFR drop per year	years of useful kidney function
7.5	3
5	5
2.5	11
1.5	19
1	29

5 to 2.5, added six years.

2.5 to 1.5 added eight years.

1.5 to 1, added ten years.

Every point or even half point you slow your decline in kidney function may add years of life to your kidneys and likely yourself as well. Imagine going from the average uneducated patient (like all of us in the beginning) to a very educated patient. The difference could be ten or twenty years of useful kidney life.

Studies suggest a 40% or 50% reduction in GFR decline may equal 70%+ longer life for your kidneys and likely you as well.

This is another reason why getting every single point of GFR improvement or every point or even half point of slowed GFR decline is so important. You have to get it just right for this to happen. Deviate from the treatment plan here at your own risk.

The diet in this book is designed to take the workload off your kidneys and cure, reduce, or treat as many comorbid conditions as possible. The hope is you will be able to slow or maybe even stop the progression of your disease. However, you may think this is impossible or maybe it's not worth trying. You don't know if it will work or not and you really don't want to go on a diet.

While I can't guarantee the diet and treatment plan will work. I can guarantee one thing.

Every treatment you don't try is guaranteed to fail.

Like our son and my own treatments, we didn't know if intensive therapy would help or not, but we knew we had to try. Not trying felt like giving up, and who can give up on a two year old? I will say this again:

Every treatment you don't try is guaranteed to fail.

You should always be under a doctor's care with no exceptions. However, the so called experts may not be so expert after all. If an "expert" tells you to give up, then maybe you need a different expert. You may want to try something your doctor has never heard of before. If that's the case, you both need to get educated. You may want to try a treatment that is not available in your state or country. Again, you and your caregivers have to get educated. We will always help and support in any way we can.

There is an attitude that as patients (or even parents) we know nothing and that we should just gracefully accept our sentence without questioning or trying every treatment option. This is bullshit, bullshit, bullshit! I was told I was "being difficult," and "I should just accept my diagnosis" at one point for seeking experimental treatments after traditional treatments failed.

Doing something different or trying hard not to die young is considered radical or extreme. I hate this idea with every fiber of my being. We, our doctors, and caregivers should be trying every option to slow or stop our disease from the day of diagnosis.

The reason for this chaos is no accepted or standardized treatment plans for incurable kidney disease. Incurable can be translated to " it's up to you to find a way."

You will find no logical reasons not to try the diet in this book and the companion book *Stopping Kidney Disease*. Go ahead and press your caregivers to get the help you need and deserve.

The diet in this book is not radical or extreme. Going on dialysis or waiting for a transplant is extreme. Thirteen people die every day in the US waiting for a transplant. The number has to be in the hundreds globally. You and I should fight anyone who tells us we should not try something new as long as we understand the risks. We have a right and a duty to try everything to slow or stop our disease. You should always be under a doctor's care, but it's fair to demand to try something new. Educating our caregivers is something we need to get used to. Educating caregivers and advocating for yourself is a key skill we all need.

In summary, the fastest dissemination of new information and ideas is going to come from those of us with a lot to lose. The people advising us have no skin in the game and little to no incentive to take a risk. Don't expect too much help with an incurable disease. Success is going to come from education on your disease and treatment options. You must take the lead in pursuing treatment options.

No one else is coming to save us; you have to save you. You have to get educated so you can make better choices and try as many treatment options as you can to live as long as you can. Your outcome will be tied directly to how educated your get and what you are willing to settle for or fight for. Fighting has a lot more upside and is a lot more fun. Don't settle just because an "expert" told you to. Do your own research, get empowered, and use facts to fight like hell.

Read *Stopping Kidney Disease* and then this book; then try it for 90 days and use your blood and urine tests to see if it works or not. If it doesn't help you, then move on to the next treatment. You should expect to see results from any treatment plan; this is no exception. If this book does not help you, then move on to the next thing.

Get educated and motivated to try to slow or stop your disease, and don't let anyone stop you. Yes, you should always be under a doctor's care at all times, but you have a right and a duty to get educated, look at all possible treatments, and try those treatments until something works.

The only way this is possible is through patient education.

CHAPTER 1

Understanding the basics or 'Kidney Factors'

Before I start, let me say again if you don't have the companion book *Stopping Kidney Disease* you may not get the references in this book. Stop here and get the companion book before continuing. The books were designed to go together. I am going to make this book short and sweet compared to *Stopping Kidney Disease* as it already covers the real research behind this diet. I can hear the sighs of relief already.

The factor approach to slowing kidney disease

In *Stopping Kidney Disease*, I listed over 20 factors that drive the progression of kidney disease. I also listed a few neutral issues and several factors that slow the progression of kidney disease.

As kidney patients, we need to change the way we think about kidney diets. Instead of managing three conditions (potassium, phosphorus, and sodium) we want to cure as many conditions as possible. The reason is every time we wrestle a test back into the normal range our odds get better.

Having potassium, phosphorus, and sodium in the normal range, but having our blood urea nitrogen(BUN), creatinine, blood pH(acidosis), inflammation markers and others above the normal range is not a victory or even good management of your disease. Our disease will still progress and our GFR will continue dropping if we go this route.

The name "Kidney Factor Eating Plan" is based on the idea that we want to treat or cure as many factors as we can (not just three) that are driving the progression of our disease. We are going to eat for our kidneys and give our kidneys a break. We want to reduce the bad factors and increase the good factors hence the "Factor" name.

By addressing the factors that drive the progression of our disease, we have the potential to slow or even stop our disease. We are going to take our foot off the gas and stop driving 100 mph toward kidney failure.

Let's list these factors to see if they are treatable by diet or not - maybe I am the crazy one?

Comorbid conditions that speed kidney disease progression.	Is diet an effective treatment?
Uremia	yes
Uremic toxins	yes
Inflammation	yes
Acidosis/Renal acid load	yes
Low serum albumin	yes
Proteinuria	yes
Sodium	yes
Phosphorus	yes
Potassium	yes
Oxidative stress	yes
Weight	yes
Hypercalcemia	yes
Hypermagnesemia	yes
Blood pressure	yes
Advanced Glycation end products (AGEs)	yes
Hyperlipidemia/Cholesterol	yes
Endothelial dysfunction	yes
Methionine restriction	yes
Heart disease	yes
Type 2 diabetes	yes
Uremic malnutrition	yes
Kwashiorkor (form of protein malnutrition)	yes
Marasmus (form of protein and calorie malnutrition)	yes
Heart disease	yes

How about a combination of diet and exercise:

Heart disease	yes
Type 2 diabetes	yes
Grip Strength	yes

We believe the following are likely improved by diet and/or diet and exercise, but we are not 100% sure yet:

Renal hypoxia	likely
Endotoxemia	unknown
Anemia	maybe
Depression/Anxiety	maybe

What drivers of kidney disease cannot be treated by a combination of diet and exercise?

Genetic diseases may not be stopped, but they may be slowed, like polycystic kidney disease.

Other health conditions/diseases outside the scope of this book.

Drugs and therapy may be required for depression and/or anxiety.

Now what about the factors that may slow disease progression: can they be treated by diet and/or exercise?

Keto acids or Keto analogues (Albutrix)	yes
Magnesium	yes
Curing comorbid conditions	yes
Curing all types of malnutrition	yes
Reducing or stopping Vascular Calcification	yes
Reducing or eliminating supplemental calcium	yes

Okay, so maybe I am not so crazy after all.

93% of conditions can be improved by diet and or a combination of diet and exercise. As you can see, the idea that we can manage only potassium, phosphorus, and sodium is a completely insane and a stone age approach to managing kidney disease unless your goal is dialysis or a transplant. If this approach died today, it wouldn't be soon enough. Yes, it is the standard advice in 2019, but it is still pure insanity. Keep reading; I will prove this to you in the next chapter. I will keep saying it: the three symptom approach is 50+ years old and has to go.

Now, let's take a recipe from a current kidney diet textbook. A 2004 edition of *Nutritional Management of Renal Disease*, 2nd edition (one of the books used to train medical professionals) recommends food like this for lunch:

2 slices of white bread

2 oz chicken

2 tsp mayonnaise

Lettuce leaf

½ medium pear

1 can of regular soda

A white bread chicken sandwich and a Coke, really? This logic is still being taught in 2019. This recipe could be any number of recipes that contain certain grains, chicken, beef, fish, pork, or cheese. These foods virtually guarantee malnutrition as our disease progresses.

I get recipes forwarded to me from patients of dialysis clinics or other nephrology related email lists every week. They all contain the same qualities: high protein, high acid load, and little to no antioxidants or vitamin-rich foods in an attempt to lower phosphorus, sodium, and potassium.

Let's go back to our list of factors that drive kidney disease progression and look at these recommendations:

Do traditional kidney diets really help us on the factors that drive kidney disease?

Uremia	no
Uremic toxins	no
Inflammation	no
Acidosis/Renal acid load	no
Low serum albumin	no
Proteinuria	no
Sodium	yes

Phosphorus	yes
Potassium	yes
Oxidative stress	no
Weight	maybe
Hypercalcemia	no
Hypermagnesemia	no
Blood pressure	no
Advanced Glycation end products (AGEs)	no
Hyperlipidemia/Cholesterol	no
Endothelial dysfunction	no
Methionine restriction	no
Heart disease	no
Type 2 diabetes	no
Uremic malnutrition	no
Kwashiorkor (form of protein malnutrition)	no
Marasmus (form of protein and calorie malnutrition)	no
Heart disease	no

10% to 15% of the list of conditions are improved by traditional kidney diets. This leaves 85% to 90% of factors untreated or unmanaged. We are not treating the majority of factors that may speed or slow disease progression. For those of us with skin in the game, treating three factors is like putting a bandaid on a broken leg. Remember, the analogy of treating three out of ten broken bones?

We need to call traditional kidney diets what they are: out of date, inadequate, flawed, apathetic, lazy, assembly lines for billion dollar dialysis clinics or whatever words you want to use.

The following chart may help explain what happens to us on traditional kidney diets.

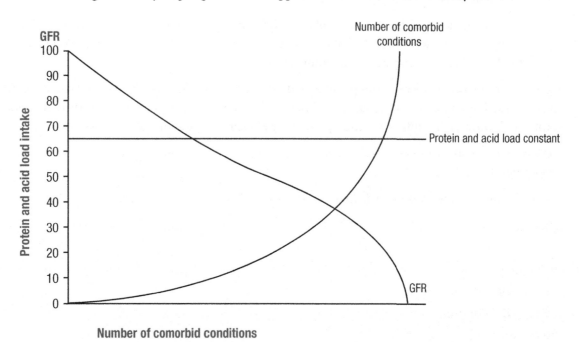

Protein and renal acid load remain the same throughout the disease. As your kidney function declines, the number of conditions increase in number and severity, first slowing, then more dramatically. In many ways, we succumb to the number of comorbid conditions caused by kidney disease. Traditional kidney diets don't lower protein or acid load or anything except for phosphorus, potassium, and sodium no matter what your GFR is in most cases. This is the road to hell.

How about specially made low-protein food products like low-protein cheese or spaghetti? These are used to lower dietary protein. These were recommended to me in the late 1990s, and I have tried most of them.

Check out the ingredients in low-protein cheese product:

Water, food starch, partially hydrogenated soybean oil, modified food starch, milk protein concentrate, salt, natural flavor, sodium phosphate, stabilizers (xanthan, locust bean, guar gum), sorbic acid, lactic acid, artificial colors.

I can't even say what effect these foods will have on us. Is it even food? Nothing on the ingredient list looks like a real food, and salt and phosphorus are added as well.

Let's go back to our list again and see if manufactured low-protein foods help kidney patients?

Uremia	yes
Uremic toxins	yes
Inflammation	no
Acidosis/Renal acid load	no
Low serum albumin	no
Proteinuria	no
Sodium	no
Phosphorus	no
Potassium	yes
Oxidative stress	no
Weight	maybe
Hypercalcemia	no
Hypermagnesemia	no
Blood pressure	no
Advanced Glycation end products (AGEs)	maybe
Hyperlipidemia/Cholesterol	no
Endothelial dysfunction	no
Methionine restriction	no
Heart disease	no
Type 2 diabetes	no
Uremic malnutrition	no
Kwashiorkor (form of protein malnutrition)	no
Marasmus (form of protein and calorie malnutrition)	no
Heart disease	no

Low protein diets address only 10% to 15% of your issues just like traditional kidney diets. This is one of the primary reasons low or very low protein diets have a mixed track record. We are still not treating the underlying or comorbid conditions. In this case, we lowered protein but consumed something from a science experiment. We got calories but not much else. No antioxidants, fiber, vitamins, and so on. We treated one factor: protein.

Three weeks ago, the news headlines were filled with the fact that ultra-processed foods decrease our life span by 15%. Ultra-processed foods have calories, added sugars and fats, chemicals, artificial colors and flavors, and a long or almost eternal shelf life. These foods have little to no fiber, antioxidants, vitamins, minerals, etc.

This week, the news is bad diet is now the biggest killer in the world. We get lots of calories, but not enough vitamins and nutrients. We don't get enough fruits, veggies, whole grains, nuts and seeds.

Kidney disease disproportionately affects low income families. One of the theories is that these families are more likely to buy cheaper foods or ultra-processed foods. Over time, the stress of these foods and lack of nutrition leads to disease. These foods are high in salt, phosphorus, added sugars, and other ingredients that are bad for us.

Do we want to be eating the absolute lowest cost ingredients with added chemicals that make it last forever? Convenience is nice, but our lives and loved ones are nicer.

Objections

I get a few objections on kidney diets. The main objections are cost and time.

Quotes like "It costs too much to eat healthy, so this is not a realistic option for many people." This is an absolute lie. It costs less than fast food averaging less than $3.00 per meal.

To address this objection I have included the estimated cost for each meal. It's cheaper than McDonalds or other fast food and cheaper than buying prepared foods.

Enough said.

The next objection is time. You will have to prepare your own meals. This does take some time but not much. Would you rather take an extra 10-30 minutes per day or eat the cheapest crap available? I hated cooking but have grown to enjoy it. It's now part of my routine. Time is a valid objection but only a very small one.

Objections from caregivers are compliance related. The compliance rates for patients following special diets is very low. Even the most optimistic estimates have dietary compliance around 20% to 25%. The normal range is 10% to 15%. There are many reasons why this is a sad fact. I have lost a lot of sleep trying to find a way to address this issue. Diets and food are emotional things for some reason. Antabuse is a pill given to alcoholics. Antabuse makes you sick if you drink alcohol. If we had a form of antabuse for kidney patients, we could get 70%+ compliance with kidney diets.

You won't get sick today if you eat food bad for your heart and kidney. You will get sick someday just not today. We have to connect the dots.

One partial solution is crowdsourcing recipes and meal plans. Our goal is to make every recipe in this book a winner and one that most people are happy to eat. The truth is some will be winners and others will be losers.

Later you will be asked to go *www.stoppingkidneydisease.com/recipeinput* to fill out a survey on the best and worst recipes. We will throw out the bad ones and keep the good ones. Get on the email list and you will get the new ones for free. Over time, the goal is to have the greatest recipes for kidney patients rated by kidney patients. Better recipes and meal plans should improve compliance rates. A diet that is cheap, easy, fun and a little decadent while still be healthy and might improve compliance.

Here is my rebuttal to all objections: Give my plan a faithful 90 days and compare the results with your plan or any other treatment plan. If you get better results with your plan or another plan, you should stick with it. If you get better results from my plan, then stick with it. Go with the facts from your blood and urine tests. Your blood and urine tests trump all manner of theory. It doesn't matter what you use to get better. Getting better is the real goal, not using a certain method or plan.

Same answer for your dietician, nutrition or doctor: Try my plan for 90 days and then try their plan for 90 days, and stick with the one that benefits you and your kidneys the most.

Whatever you do, don't blindly accept watching your kidney function decline each year without trying everything.

What we eat and drink today determines how fast our kidneys will decline (or not decline) over the upcoming years. It is that simple.

Back to the "Factors"

We are going to treat as many of these factors as we can and see what happens 90 days later. This is a simple, direct, and most of all, measurable approach to kidney disease management. We aren't going to guess if this plan works, we are going to use facts to guide our decisions.

Now, you can see why patients are getting such different results from this diet and treatment plan. We are going to try to treat 20+ factors that drive our disease, not just three.

You need to embrace the changes so you can find out if you can stop or slow your disease. I am still in partial remission 11 years later. I am still on a form of the diet today. I am sure many of you will do even better than I did.

I still worry that I could fall out of remission any day. Once your kidneys are damaged, these diets are part of your life forever. That's another reason we need to improve the recipes. Go back to normal eating and suffer the consequences. I tried this after remission and things starting going badly again. Learn from my mistakes—let me be your crash test dummy. It's the one thing I am really good at. I call my current status: "voluntary remission."

You can voluntarily slow your disease progression, maybe even stop it, and get healthier as well. It's voluntary because you have to do your part. And yes, you can also voluntarily drive 100 mph toward dialysis as well.

My hope is you will try everything to slow or stop your disease and be successful whether it is with this plan or another. Remember, the longer you wait to treat your disease, the harder it will be.

CHAPTER 2

Saving yourself and 10,000 other patients from malnutrition

This chapter is about something that was a dietary atom bomb for me and generated a lot of questions from fellow patients. It hit me like a ton of bricks when I finally put two and two together.

I am going to start with a study about albumin and saving the lives of thousands of kidney patients each year.

Study 2.1   Revisiting mortality predictability of serum albumin in the dialysis population: time dependency, longitudinal changes, and population-attributable fraction.1

Time-varying hypoalbuminemia predicts all-cause and CV death differently from fixed measures of serum albumin in MHD patients. An increase in serum albumin over time is associated with better survival independent of baseline serum albumin or other MICS surrogates. If this association is causal, an intervention that could increase serum albumin >3.8 g/dl might reduce the number of MHD deaths in the USA by approximately 10,000 annually. Nutritional interventions examining benefits of increasing serum albumin in MHD patients are urgently needed.

Ok, this research was speaking about dialysis patients only. If the number is 10,000 a year for dialysis, then it must be in the hundreds of thousands for all kidney patients. We have no way to know an exact number, but the number could be in the tens of thousands in the United States alone because over 20 million people are affected by kidney disease. Globally, the number has got to be over 100,000 people who might be saved by better nutrition each year.

Let me state this even clearer: Protein malnutrition is killing us because we don't treat the underlying causes.

Albumin is covered extensively in Stopping Kidney Disease chapter four. For those who have not read chapter four, albumin is a protein in your blood. The value of albumin is widely debated as a diagnostic tool. Is it a nutrition, acidosis, or inflammation marker. There is some debate on this. My previous nephrologist told me "Don't worry about albumin, it doesn't really tell you anything about nutrition." Wrong, just plain wrong.

I am going to worry and worry a lot. See the next study to see why I was so worried.

Study 2.2   Uremic malnutrition is a predictor of death independent of inflammatory status.

CONCLUSION:

The nutritional status of CHD patients predicts mortality independent of concomitant presence or absence of inflammatory response. Prevention of, and timely intervention to treat uremic malnutrition by suitable means are necessary independent of the presence and/or therapy of inflammation in terms of improving clinical outcomes in CHD patients.

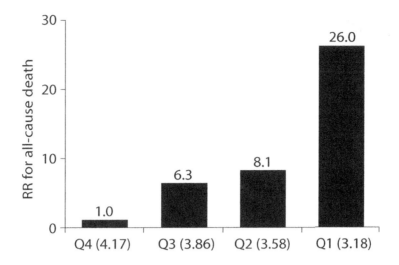

Relative risk for all-cause death according to quartiles of mean serum albumin during the study period. Patients with serum albumin concentrations ≤3.18 g/dL were 26 times more likely to die of any cause compared with those with serum albumin concentrations ≥4.17 g/dL. $P < 0.001$ Q2, 3, and 4 vs. Q1.

As the chart shows, your risk of dying may be 26 times higher depending on your albumin level, even after inflammation is taken out of the picture. There's no need to debate if albumin is important anymore. Hundreds of studies agree on the value of albumin as an accurate and strong mortality indicator.

I was not just worried, I was freaking out, as my albumin was 1.7 mg/dl at the worst. Almost 50% lower than 3.8 g/dl. The normal range for albumin is 3.5 to 5.5 mg/dl. However, we know our odds get worse if you drop below 4.1 g/dl.

```
                          DATE    09/02/98
                          TIME    1415
                          DAY      WED

        PROCEDURE


        MISCELLANEOUS GENERAL CHEM
        TOTAL PROTEIN              3.8L
        SPE ALBUMIN               1.70L
        SPE A-1                    0.20
        SPE A-2                    1.00H
        SPE BETA                   0.60
        SPE GAMMA                 0.40L
        SPE INTERP              FOOTNOTE£
              09/02/98 1415
```

I had a 60% chance of dying over the next 30 days according to some research. For the record, at the time I was eating high protein (100+ grams), high acid load, low antioxidant and low nutrient value and getting plenty of calories. I was single and working 50+ hours a week eating junk.

Today, 21 years later, my albumin is more than 130% higher in the low 4's and has been for a decade. So don't tell me you can't raise or treat low albumin. I promise you can, but you have to treat the underlying issues first.

Unique to kidney patients

Uremic Malnutrition is a form of malnutrition specific to kidney patients. Over time, we lose the ability to properly metabolize or process dietary protein. It looks like this happens when our GFR drops below 60ish. This is an educated guess based on several studies. We are eating enough dietary protein to meet our needs but still have low protein levels as expressed by serum albumin measurements. A number of factors work independently and together to reduce our ability to metabolize or process dietary protein. We can no longer synthesize or make needed proteins and proteins our body makes or digests are degraded before they can be used by our bodies.

These factors are:

Acidosis

Uremia, uremic toxins

Oxidative stress

Inflammation

Proteinuria, which is losing or "leaking" protein in our urine

And likely a few more we don't know about.

Atom bomb time

Simple question: Can we save those 10,000 patients a year using traditional kidney diets?

Answer: No, traditional kidney diets are actually causing this form of malnutrition.

Traditional kidney diets keep piling on the very things that our blood tests are telling us we shouldn't be eating. As our kidney function and ability to properly process protein drops, protein intake stays the same despite falling kidney function. This results in a faster disease progression and higher percentages of malnutrition.

Let's go a step further: Are traditional kidney diets causing low serum albumin levels? The answer is (hear me screaming) "YES!"

How can the diets that are supposed to be good for us actually be bad for us?

Chicken, beef, fish, pork, cheese, and many grains have a few things in common:

1. They have a very high renal acid load, the highest of any food as a group causing acidosis.

2. They produce the highest levels of nitrogen and waste products causing uremia and contributing to uremic toxins. This shows in your blood urea nitrogen (BUN) and creatinine levels outside the normal range.

3. They contain an insignificant amount of antioxidants or none at all but create free radicals or oxidative stress.

4. Red meat may contribute to inflammation; others are unknown. However, the combination of high acid load, high waste workload, and no antioxidants contribute to inflammation.

5. Proteinuria can be reduced by reducing protein intake, inflammation, oxidative stress, and uremia, not increasing these factors.

Meat is recommended due to the high biological value, which means these foods contain all of the essential amino acids. This part makes sense for healthy people. Essential amino acids are the ones your body cannot produce. However, eating this form of protein virtually guarantees low serum albumin levels by contributing strongly to acidosis, uremia, inflammation, advanced glycation end products, oxidative stress, proteinuria, and so on.

As our kidney function expressed as GFR drops, so does our albumin level. Our GFR levels tend to track our albumin levels. As our ability to process protein drops we keep piling on those factors that cause malnutrition, our GFR and albumin levels drop because our bodies can't handle the workload any more. Many of the factors we need to limit or stop all together are a key part of traditional kidney diets.

A continuing decline in GFR should be expected with these diets. It can't be any other way; there is no other possible outcome with these diets. One look at your blood tests will confirm this theory is correct.

It doesn't matter whether you think albumin is a nutritional or inflammation marker or whatever kind of marker. The academic argument doesn't matter; what matters is our risk of dying and the speed of disease progression.

Albumin levels are a window into the war going on inside our body. Albumin levels take into account dietary intake, inflammation, acidosis, oxidative stress and so on. We know that no matter what your albumin level is today, your odds improve if your albumin is rising. Your odds get worse if your albumin is falling, no matter how high your levels are today.

The dietary atom bomb for me was threefold:

1. Traditional kidney diets were causing the problem I was trying to solve like falling serum albumin, continued decline in GFR, and blood tests outside the normal range.

2. These same conditions could be improved or cured by a diet that addressed the underlying conditions causing malnutrition.

3. The product I needed to improve was not available in the US, and the overseas version was going to kill me via heart disease due to a combination of my family history and high amounts of supplemental calcium.

We easily treat something that may kill thousands of patients each year, but we have not been able to. This was an atom bomb for me for me personally. I was doing everything I was told, but my disease was still progressing and no one seemed to care.

If low albumin is treatable, why are so many people dying each year? Simple: kidney diets and treatment plans have not progressed in 50 years.

The effects of diet and malnutrition affect us down to a cellular level (see the next study). Protein-energy wasting is a term used to describe protein malnutrition like uremic malnutrition and similar conditions.

Study 2.3   Protein-Energy Wasting and Mortality in Chronic Kidney Disease

ABSTRACT:

Protein-energy wasting (PEW) is common in patients with chronic kidney disease (CKD) and is associated with an increased death risk from cardiovascular diseases. However, while even minor renal dysfunction is an independent predictor of adverse cardiovascular prognosis, PEW becomes clinically manifest at an advanced stage, early before or during the dialytic stage. Mechanisms causing loss of muscle protein and fat are complex and not always associated with anorexia, but are linked to several abnormalities that stimulate protein degradation and/or decrease protein synthesis. In addition, data from experimental CKD indicate that uremia specifically blunts the regenerative potential in skeletal muscle, by acting on muscle stem cells. In this discussion recent findings regarding the mechanisms responsible for malnutrition and the increase in cardiovascular risk in CKD patients are discussed. During the course of CKD, the loss of kidney excretory and metabolic functions proceed together with the activation of pathways of endothelial damage, inflammation, acidosis, alterations in insulin signaling and anorexia which are likely to orchestrate net protein catabolism and the PEW syndrome.

Some notes from this study:

> Uremia blunts the ability to build muscle by acting on stem cells.

> Muscle loss/Sarcopenia is common in kidney patients.

> Multiple factors like inflammation and acidosis are also related.

Other studies which are not listed here show that in addition to affecting muscle growth, uremia affects stem cells in bone marrow and wound healing, and this can happen early in kidney disease.

All of the factors in this study can be changed by lowering dietary protein intake.

This form of malnutrition affects us down to a stem cell level! This means when your blood urea nitrogen (BUN) and creatinine tests are above the normal range, you will start being affected. No, you will not have a clinical diagnosis of uremia, but you can bet you are going to start suffering the cumulative consequences over time.

Again, the dietary atom bomb for me was that the nutritionist and doctor's advice at the time made my malnutrition issues get worse, not better. My test results were telling me I was doing the wrong things, but I still blindly followed their advice. Yes, my phosphorus, potassium, and sodium got better, but my GFR, blood urea nitrogen, creatinine, and amount of protein in my urine kept getting worse. Hmm, maybe something is wrong? I can't be the first one to see or observe this?

We should be lowering protein and acid load to compensate for our reduced kidney function, but we don't.

Ok, this book series is about education, so now let's lay down some real understanding of malnutrition issues for kidney patients before leaving this chapter.

Understanding the difference between intake and processing malnutrition

Understanding this difference is key to understanding your current blood and urine tests. It is also key to understanding why your current diet is not working. I am going to use the word "intake" to describe malnutrition based on dietary intake and "processing" to describe when your body cannot properly process dietary protein. It's important to understand these are very different problems.

Let's start with the two types of intake malnutrition:

> Kwashiorkor is a dietary protein deficiency with adequate calories. We are not eating enough protein to meet our needs.

> Marasmus is a protein- and calorie-deficient diet. We are not eating enough of anything to meet our needs.

These conditions happen if your diet is deficient in either calories, protein, or both for a long enough time period. A few days won't matter but weeks will start to matter. The good news is that both of these are treatable by increasing protein, calories, or both. I am not going to spend more time on these as the next one is a biggie for us.

Uremic malnutrition is the other form we have been talking about, and this is a processing problem, not an intake problem. You can't treat uremic malnutrition like an intake problem. You must treat it as what it is: a processing problem caused by putting too much workload on your kidneys. That's the problem with traditional kidney diets. These diets act as if we don't have a processing problem despite our numbers being outside the normal range and our GFR dropping.

Another way to look at this issue is comorbid conditions. Comorbid conditions are issues that are associated with our main disease or go with a disease. A way to look at kidney disease is death by comorbid conditions. Kidney disease is not the cause of death. The cause of death is one of the many comorbid conditions caused by kidney disease. Traditional kidney diets do little to address comorbid conditions like acidosis and high nitrogen and creatinine levels.

Traditional kidney diets trade causing some comorbid conditions while trying to manage others. Treating three comorbid conditions while causing three or four more comorbid conditions is not the goal of any kidney patient. We should always be working to cure every comorbid condition we have. The accumulation of these conditions is what kills us in the end. The idea that accumulating or contributing to more conditions is the best approach needs to die.

How much is too much protein?

How do you know you are eating too much dietary protein?

It's simple. Your blood urea nitrogen (BUN) and/or creatinine levels are higher than the upper limit. This is not rocket science. If your BUN level is above 20 mg/dL or (7.1 mmol/L) and/or your creatinine level is greater than **1.2** mg/dl, your kidneys are screaming that you are eating more protein than they can safely process. You have a black and white factual answer right in front of you.

If your numbers are higher than the normal range, you are eating more dietary protein in a 24-hour period than your kidneys and body can effectively process in 24 hours. You are overloading your kidneys with work and doing this will increase the rate and speed that you develop more comorbid conditions and speed kidney disease progression.

Combine this with serum albumin below 4.1 g/dl and you have or are in the beginning stages of uremic malnutrition. Your risks start to skyrocket. To be clear, you will not meet a clinical diagnosis with these numbers, but I couldn't care less about a name or technical diagnosis anymore. I care that my odds of dying start rising dramatically when I drop below 4.1 g/dl. We also know that creatinine and BUN levels higher than the normal range are the earliest stages of uremia. Your doctor will not mention this as you don't meet the clinical definition, but you do need to care at this stage.

Your body and kidneys are screaming for you to change your ways. You just need to listen and heed their advice. Your kidneys opinion (via blood test) on your current diet outrank anyone's opinion. Your body, all the way to the stem cell level, is going to start to be affected. Take a second to think about this. All the way down to the building blocks of our bodies are affected.

I was told to reduce my sodium, potassium, and phosphorus and eat more protein when my serum albumin was 1.7 g/dl. This advice turned out to be wrong, dead wrong. In fact, they could not be more wrong if they tried. This is the exact opposite of what I needed to do to get better. The belief that eating more protein will solve the problem or is helpful in some way is a complete lack of understanding of protein metabolism in kidney patients and the different types of malnutrition.

What do we need to do?

Study 2.4   Management of protein-energy wasting in non-dialysis-dependent chronic kidney disease: reconciling low protein intake with nutritional therapy

CONCLUSIONS

PEW (protein energy wasting) is a powerful predictor of outcomes over the entire range of CKD and often can be alleviated by ensuring adequate protein and energy intake (37). Conversely, uncontrolled high protein intakes can have deleterious consequences, including biochemical imbalances such as hyperkalemia and hyperphosphatemia, and worsening oxidative stress, altered endothelial function, nitric oxide production, insulin resistance, glomerular hyperfiltration, and uremic symptoms. Dietary interventions for PEW must both ensure adequate intakes of protein and energy and avoid deleterious effects of high protein intakes. These seemingly contradictory goals can only be achieved with careful attention to both the quantity and quality of ingested proteins and to the intake of other nutrients. Potential strategies to achieve these goals include supplementing the usual (or low) amount of protein in the diet with essential nutrients or supplements that are specifically designed for CKD patients (75) and/or prevention of the deleterious side effects of high dietary protein intake (eg, binder medications and alkali). The effectiveness and safety of these strategies at improving patient outcomes will need to be confirmed in future studies.

Note: This study sums it up nicely: We are managing contradictory goals, balancing between too little and too much protein while we are trying to treat multiple comorbid conditions. This can be done with a little practice, record keeping, and the motivation to follow a plan.

We need specific drugs or foods to address our exact problems and we need to understand our exact protein needs. We want to walk a fine line between getting too much protein and not getting enough protein. Both are bad for us.

One more study to think about:

Study 2.5   Malnutrition in Chronic Kidney Disease and Relationship to Quality of Life

ABSTRACT:

Protein-energy malnutrition and impaired quality of life are the most important complications of chronic kidney disease. Several factors such as inadequate nutrient intake due to anorexia, metabolic acidosis and chronic inflammation can contribute to malnutrition of patients with chronic kidney disease. Risk of hospitalization and mortality is inversely correlated to nutritional markers. Quality of life of patients with chronic kidney disease is worse than that of the healthy controls. Besides chronic kidney disease itself, the impairment in quality of life can be related to its complications such as anemia, malnutrition, as well as comorbid conditions, such as diabetes and cardiovascular disease. While much of the data about the relationship between the patient's nutritional state and quality of life have been obtained in dialysis patients, there is convincing evidence that malnutrition begins earlier in chronic kidney disease and affects the self-perceived quality of life of the patients. It has been shown that quality of life is an important factor that predicts morbidity and mortality. To improve the quality of life, patients with chronic kidney disease should be referred to nephrology units without delay, so that complications and comorbid conditions could be managed appropriately.

A few notes from this study:

Protein energy malnutrition (PEW) is one of the most important factors for us to address.

Risk of hospitalization and mortality is inversely correlated to nutritional markers.

Malnutrition begins early, for me is was stage 3.

Repeat: Our risk of hospitalization and mortality is inversely correlated to nutritional markers.

A good rule of thumb is when your GFR drops below 65, bad things start happening with traditional diets or traditional kidney diets.

Depending on the study you read, 10% to 70% of hemodialysis patients and 18% to 51% of ambulatory peritoneal dialysis patients have some form of malnutrition. Malnutrition typically starts in stage three and then picks up steam from there. Again, A GFR in the 60's or below is where bad things start to happen.

Studies suggest malnutrition is around 40% to 70% in kidney patients not on dialysis. It's clear malnutrition is affecting most of us.

We can change the outcomes for you and me.

There is no reason whatsoever that a kidney patient should suffer from malnutrition in 2019. The only reasons are apathy or lack of understanding.

In 2018 and 2019, Albutrix became available in the US and other countries. Albutrix is a specially designed low nitrogen protein food to help us raise albumin levels, provide all essential amino acids, and not contribute to the underlying issues we are trying to cure. This is the big key. We need protein supplements that don't contribute to the very issues that increase our risks or the speed of kidney and heart disease progression.

We worked for years to ensure Albutrix helped treat the underlying conditions and not cause more problems like traditional solutions.

For example, Albutrix has:

1. Negative acid load so we don't contribute to or help reduce acidosis
2. Coated pills mask the bad taste of protein powders and liquids
3. Pills are also the most convenient form for busy lives and increases compliance by making things easier
4. Lowest amounts of supplemental calcium again to reduce vascular calcification and mortality risks
5. Suggested servings contain less than the recommended daily amounts (RDA) to increase safety
6. Acts as phosphorus binder to reduce phosphorus levels
7. 100% Ornithine free
8. Very low amounts of sodium, phosphorus, and potassium
9. Easy to measure dosage by using pills vs powders or liquids
10. Specific nutrition to address each stage of kidney disease. Stage 5 patients have different needs than Stage 3 patients. Past solutions were all designed for stage 5 patients
11. Amino acid profile is based on providing the RDA of all essential amino acids after dietary intake is accounted for
12. Magnesium to reduce vascular calcification, reduce supplemental calcium and reduce inflammation. Patients with high magnesium levels have a survival advantage.

Albutrix has a lot is going on underneath the hood by design. We have to do a few things to be really successful with protein supplementation. I had five main goals:

1. Provide protein nutrition, but do not create or contribute to more or accelerated comorbid conditions like acidosis and vascular calcification(the number one killer of kidney patients).

2. Provide protein nutrition and attempt to reduce, lessen or treat as many comorbid conditions at the same time.

3. Provide protein nutrition to raise albumin levels while not violating #1 and #2.

4. Provide protein nutrition with the lowest possible nitrogen load to allow a higher or more flexible protein restriction(aka easier diet).

5. Make it as easy as possible on patients.

These goals required us to spend over a year learning how to make materials needed to hit these goals. The materials were not available in the global markets, so we had to develop techniques, procedures and production to make these materials. We also had to learn from the failures of the past 30 years. Albutrix is the only low nitrogen protein food in the world using these materials.

So In real life, a lot of things have to happen for patients to be successful on low protein diets using a protein supplement. This is why low protein diets have such a mixed track record. Things can get worse if we are not careful or we swap one condition for another or add to the number of conditions we have trying to get protein nutrition.

I have tried to address as many of the factors as I could. The outcomes so far have been better than I ever expected. It is unreasonable to think every single kidney patients can benefit, but the results so far have greatly exceeded my expectations.

We did something else to increase access regardless of where you live. Albutrix ships free to almost any country in the world from **www.albutrix.com**. Why does Albutrix ship free worldwide?

I did this because I was denied access to treatment because of where I lived. I desperately needed something like Albutrix when my albumin numbers were low. No one should ever have to choose between being a criminal and trying to stop a deadly disease. In our first month, we shipped to nine countries who would not have access otherwise. Again, patient-to-patient is the fastest way we are going to help each other. If you are a patient trying to live longer and better, we are on your team regardless of where you live.

I personally view Albumin levels as one of the most important measurements for us.

Remember this:

Albumin rising = outlook is getting better

Albumin falling = outlook is getting worse

Let me say it again, for good measure. Protein malnutrition should be a thing of the past. The only reason it should exist today is if you make a conscious choice to be malnourished or choose to ignore your test results.

In summary:

Traditional kidney diets suck. I don't have an emoji for "the finger," or I would have used it for my summary.

The diet you are on may be doing more harm than good. Just check your creatinine, blood urea nitrogen (BUN), and albumin levels over time if you don't believe me. If you are getting worse, your question has been answered.

Go to **www.albutrix.com** to find out more on Albutrix—a modern low nitrogen protein food for kidney patients by kidney patients.

What is the KDA?

KDA stands for kidney daily amount. RDA stands for recommended daily amount. I copied this idea for the nutritional information in this book. This is something I made up (it's not an official name).

We are going to use KDA to describe the daily amount of something you need for your kidneys to treat as many factors as we can. KDA is something I made up years ago for myself. KDA is a way to use a standard nutrition label, like we are used to seeing on food, to give dietary information.

It will look something like this:

Nutrition Facts	
Serving Size	Entire Recipe
Amount Per Serving	
Calories	**400**
	Kidney Friendly % DV*
Total Fat 3g	4%
Saturated Fat 1.5g	8%
Trans Fat 0g	
Cholesterol 0mg	0%
Total Carbohydrate 79g	29%
Dietary Fiber 9g	30%
Total Sugars 8g	
Includes 0g Added Sugar	0%
Protein 8g	
Sodium 25mg	1%
Potassium 260mg	7%
Phosphorus 95mg	8%
ORAC 15955	53%
Polyphenols 1165mg	117%
AGE	VERY LOW
PRAL	0.4
Dietary Nitrates	HIGH

* The % Daily Value (DV) tells you how much a nutrient in a serving of food contributes to the daily kidney friendly diet. 2,000 calories a day is used for general nutrition advice.

We want to get certain foods every day so that we get 100% of our KDA or limit foods to 100% of our KDA. For example, extra polyphenols and antioxidants are fine, but we don't want extra protein, high renal acid load, AGEs, and so on.

The basics are a plant-based, low-protein, negative acid load, high-antioxidant diet using real foods. Foods with one ingredient, the actual food. We will use some foods that might be considered processed foods like plant-based milk substitutes, but we will try to keep these to a minimum.

We do have a recipe with egg whites to allow some diversity and satisfy cravings you might have. Egg whites have a much lower acid load than the whole egg. On that note, the diet is not vegan, vegetarian, paleo, or any real label. There are no food politics or agenda here. We are trying to do the workload for our kidneys with our brains and mouths and use blood tests to guide us.

Reasons for KDA

A few items on the nutrition labels are different from traditional labels, so a brief explanation is needed.

Items like total fat, cholesterol, total carbohydrates, fiber, and sugar are just like every other food label. There's no explanation needed for these items.

The ones you may not be familiar with need a little explaining. Remember, we want to treat, manage, cure, and/or reduce any and all underlying conditions that may be driving the progression of kidney and heart disease. Curing all comorbid conditions should be part of your treatment goal. As a reminder, the more comorbid conditions you have, the greater your odds of dying.

There are very important reasons why the KDA tracks issues that no other diets currently track or account for. The reasons are multiple medical studies or trials showing strong benefits to our kidneys.

First, the daily percentages are based on what we think the ideal diet should be for patients, not the traditional recommended daily amounts. For example, the estimated amount of potassium for this diet is 3,500 mg a day. You will see percentages of these numbers, like the first recipe is 4% for potassium. This is 4% of 3,500 mg, not 4% of the traditional recommended daily amount which is 4,700 mg a day. We used 3,500 mg as a middle ground. Some patients will need less and others can consume more potassium. The milligrams are included for every recipe. You will have to determine what is best for you.

The protein value is based on 30 grams a day, not the normal RDA. Your body weight will differ, but it should be easy to understand.

Next, a few terms you may not be familiar with deserve explanation.

"ORAC" stands for Oxygen Radical Absorbance Capacity or the estimated antioxidant content of a food. The value of ORAC has been debated as a tool for measuring antioxidants. We are going to use it because it's really the only tool out there right now. ORAC is likely imperfect, but usable to estimate antioxidant intake. ORAC amounts for most foods can be found via the web.

Kidney patients have much higher amounts of oxidative stress. Oxidative stress is a driver of kidney disease progression. The estimate used is 30,000 ORAC units intake per day, which is what the percentage is based on. We know that 12,000 to 15,000 units are needed to reduce mortality rates and we know that ORAC units are likely reduced with cooking or processing. A goal of 30,000 ensures we still get what is likely needed after cooking or processing. You don't have to hit 30,000 every day, but you should try at least 5 days a week. Our goal here is to stop oxidative stress from being a factor in your disease progression. The effects of antioxidants last only a few hours in your body, so you need to consume them frequently.

Polyphenols are related to ORAC in some ways. Foods high in polyphenols are usually high in antioxidants as well. However, a small amount of polyphenols occur in veggies and many fruits. In order to get enough, we need to measure polyphenols so we can steer the diet in that direction. Polyphenols help with heart health and maybe renoprotective. There are many different kinds of substances that fall under polyphenols: flavonoids, anthocyanins, and many others. Tea and coffee are the most common source in the U.S. You will see an emphasis on polyphenols in the drink section as well. Polyphenol intake may end up being a big factor in slowing disease progression. If we are really trying to get better, polyphenols intake has got to be part of our plan.

AGE stands for advanced glycation end products. *Stopping Kidney Disease* has an entire chapter devoted to AGEs. AGEs are consumed when food is seared or burned in most cases. You will see no foods that are blackened or seared here. We have a few for the grill, but they are not foods that require cooking at high heats to cook the inside like traditional meats. We also limiting fried foods as well. AGEs are another driver of kidney disease we need to avoid. Kidney diets that recommended cooked meats are making a big mistake. Accurate AGE estimates are hard to find so we are using high, low, and so on as an estimate.

PRAL or potential renal acid load is an estimate of the acid intake or acid workload we are putting on our kidneys from eating different foods. Acidosis is a major driver of kidney disease. High acid diets require our kidneys to work twice as hard as needed. Our kidneys have to process the nitrogen waste products from meats and then process the ammonia produced by our bodies to offset the acid load. Fruits and veggies (mostly green veggies) contain a natural form of bicarbonate that increases our own bicarbonate stores over time. Eating a diet with a negative acid load builds these stores of bicarbonate to offset acid intake and reduce the workload on the kidneys at the same time. Numbers above 0 indicate acid, numbers below 0 indicate alkaline. We want to consume a negative acid load for the day every day. Acidosis or acid load may turn out to be one of the strongest drivers of kidney disease progression. In most cases, acidosis can be completely treated by diet. There is really no need for sodium bicarbonate or drugs for acidosis. You can just stop eating high acid foods; it's that simple in all but the most extreme cases. Your bicarbonate levels will build slowly and studies show bicarbonate levels still rising in patients who have been using a low acid diet for 18 months. This one is mandatory for us. If you are advised to eat a high acid diet, it's wrong, dead ass wrong. The research on this is new but very strong. Traditional kidney diets don't measure acid load for a variety of reasons, but the biggest reason is they are still 50 years behind.

Dietary nitrates is last and is confusing to many people. First, you may hear nitrates are bad for you. You may see foods labeled "nitrate-free" like on a package of bacon. Nitrates as a food additive may be used to preserve or extend the shelf life of foods. Nitrates as a food additive are very controversial. We are not talking about the food additive here. We are talking about naturally occurring nitrates. When we eat naturally occurring nitrates, the saliva in our mouths convert it to nitrites. Nitrites are then absorbed into our body and converted to nitric oxide. Nitric oxide relaxes our blood vessels, which increases blood flow. We should be consuming naturally occurring nitrates regularly. Research shows that naturally occurring nitrates reduce blood pressure, may be renoprotective, and lower the risk of cardiovascular events. We also know that the renal resistive index, a measure of pressure required to move blood through the kidneys, improves with dietary nitrate consumption. We have good evidence blood pressure in our kidneys is lowered and blood flow to our kidneys is increased with nitrate consumption. We also know that a higher renal resistance index number predicts aggressive kidney disease progression. A lower index predicts a better outcome. Again, if we really want to get better, this is something we should be managing and measuring.

Accurate nitrate numbers are hard to find, so we opted for low, high, and so on.

The approach for the kidney factor diet is two fold. First, we want to cure, reduce, or manage as many bad factors as we can that speed our disease and increase the factors that may slow, or maybe stop, our disease.

The second part of this approach is the idea of a minimalist approach for diet and supplements. We know that large doses of just about anything are bad for our kidneys. Traditional vitamins are an example. Studies show that large doses of B vitamins speed progression and some kidney-related vitamins have 500% of the RDA.

Think of your kidneys like a child about to fall over carrying a heavy object. My son was four and wanted to help carry firewood on a cold day. When I turned around, he was shaking and could barely stand upright due to the weight of the logs. Your kidneys are just like my son that day. If I had added one more log, he would have fallen over.

Your kidneys are already taxed and overworked. Traditional kidney diets keep piling on the work even when all evidence shows your kidneys can't manage the current workload or weight.

One gram of protein over what you need is extra workload with no reward; one gram under can lead to protein nutrition issues. We will never get it exact. We will always be a little over or a little under and that's okay. What matters is the average over the long term.

If you are eating random diets, taking lots of vitamins and supplements (we hear this a lot), your kidneys are like a child carrying too much weight. You can't see or feel it but they are struggling with the workload. The evidence is in our blood work. When you see your blood work outside the normal range, think of your own kids or grandkids falling over because they are carrying too much weight. They are trying as hard as they can, but are just not strong enough. Piling on work due to ignorance and lack of education about our kidneys and our disease is expected when we first get diagnosed. Everything is overwhelming during this period. However, the idea that the right thing to do is to continue to pile on workload when our kidneys can't handle the current workload is plain crazy. It's crazy because everything points to a faster progression of kidney and heart disease.

We want to put the absolute lowest workload possible on our kidneys. This is how we get better. We don't get better by piling on the factors that speed the progression of our disease. This is a truth and fact you need to understand.

If anyone tells you to eat a high-acid, high-protein, low-antioxidant diet that is not heart-healthy, they are not helping you. Education is the theme in this book series and the goal is to educate you. Faster progress will be made if patients can make good decisions over the long term. If you are not sure on an issue you are facing, do the research or reach out to us. We can't always help, but sometimes we can.

The bottom line is educated patients live longer and better lives because they are able to make better decisions on a daily basis.

Diet basics

The recommended daily amount of protein (from all sources) is 0.8 grams per kg of body weight. To start our diet, we are going to spit this 50/50. (0.4 grams of protein from dietary sources and another 0.4 grams of protein per kg from low nitrogen protein foods like Albutrix.)

We are starting at 0.4 grams per kg as we can still eat healthy foods given this restriction. When we drop to 0.3 grams per kg, it gets a little harder to eat real foods most of the time.

Let's go through the basic daily initial dietary goals or the KDA's.

Limit these bad factors to:

Dietary protein	0.4 grams per kg of body weight
Sodium	2,200 mg per day
Plant-based phosphorus	1,200 mg per day
Potassium	3,500 mg per day or your personal limit
AGEs	Very low or no AGEs estimate
Renal acid load	Net negative acid load for the day
Supplemental calcium intake	As little as possible, or 1 gram of total calcium per day from all sources, diet and supplements.
Saturated fats	Low intake

Increase these good factors to:

Keto acids (Albutrix)	Dosage equal to dietary protein shortfall
	One pill equals approximately four grams of dietary protein
Magnesium intake	Keep in the high end normal range
Antioxidants (ORAC)	30,000+ per day
Polyphenols	1+ gram(s) per day
Dietary Nitrates	150 mg+
Fiber	30+ grams
Heart-healthy	Eliminate foods that are not heart-healthy
Exercise	5 days a week - get with the program

I know this is a lot, but we are going to do the work for you to make it easier. If you can read a nutrition label on any food product, you are in good shape.

This kind of diet can feel like juggling while riding a unicycle on a tightrope over a shark tank, but I have done the work for you. There is nothing to fear.

Note: We can't say "anti-inflammatory" as no standard exists for this measurement. No anti-inflammatory scale has been proven. Foods high in antioxidants tend to be anti-inflammatory, but I left this out because I have no way to accurately measure it.

Everyone will have to customize the diet and meal plans to their current situation and tastes. These plans will get you off to a great start.

At the end of the book we will combine meals for you and total the amounts for the day to give you some ideas and suggestions.

Please read the treatment plan sections of *Stopping Kidney Disease* before going forward.

CHAPTER 4

Make it easy on yourself: a few tips before you start

I am not going to write much about cooking basics. I am not a good cook by any standard, and 100% of readers are adults who know their way around a kitchen and have been preparing meals for decades. However, I did want to make some observations about this diet that may help you. If something special is required, we will note in the recipe. These tips may help you along the way.

Keeping track is mandatory.

First, the only way this treatment plan works is if you keep track of the numbers. If your diet is random, then your results will be random as well. Half-assed efforts will get half-assed results. There's no way around this fact. Remember, the mantra "Moderation kills" and Garbage in, Garage out (GIGO); we are battling a disease, so keep track. It's the only way you are going to be able to adjust your diet after your first set of blood tests. In a way, this is your own personal clinical trial.

You can't correct your diet 90 days from now if you don't know what you were eating!

There are two ways to keep track. First, write down everything and measure everything. This is pretty easy to do but takes a little time.

Second is to eat the same meals or same daily meal plans frequently so you memorize what the nutrition numbers are and you don't have to think about it. Later in the book we will total these for you.

Most of us eat the same food frequently. Very few of us eat something different three times a day, seven days a week. If you are good at note-taking and disciplined about measuring and writing things down, then great.

But if you're like me, you are lucky to know what day it is. Eating the same meals frequently is the best strategy. Eating the same breakfast may sound boring, but it's the easiest way to stay on the plan. My best success was when I was in brain dead zombie autopilot mode where I ate the same foods and meals over and over again.

Pick two or three breakfasts, lunches, and dinners, plus a snack or two that you like and fit your needs and forget about the rest for a while. This is the way to dominate the diet plan. After a few days, weeks or months, make a few changes, but keep it to things you like and will eat without a gun to your head.

For a while, keep it super simple and where you can't fail. You will get the hang of it after a while, but don't put pressure on yourself. I think this is very important for the first 90 days.

Let me repeat this again: Pick a few meals you like and then don't think about or look up alternatives for 90 days.

This is the way to dominate the diet and treatment plan.

What you need to know about breakfasts, Sundays, and dessert

My personal experience is these diets are won and lost at breakfast, Sundays, and dessert. Let me explain:

My go-to breakfast is ⅓ cup low-sugar Craisins (cranberries), ¼ cup pecans, and a piece of fruit like an apple, pear, cutie (small tangerine), berries, or whatever is in the house, and two cups of coffee with soy creamer (no protein kind).

It's fast, and takes about two minutes to prepare by measuring and throwing everything in a bowl, zip-top bag, or plastic to-go container. I can take in the car, train, or wherever I am going. I can eat it now, later, or graze at my desk.

Let's look at the nutrition info:

Dried cranberries	10,000 ORAC or antioxidants and zero protein
Pecans	8,500 ORAC for ¼ cup, 2.5 grams of protein
Apple	4,500 ORAC and 1 gram of protein
Coffee	2,500 ORAC per cup or 5,000 total, no protein

There's a total of 28,000 ORAC or antioxidant count and around 3.5 to 4 grams of protein. It has lots of fiber, polyphenols, nuts for heart health, and so on. I have almost hit my antioxidant count for the day, and I used up only four grams of protein and still have 26 grams to use up later in the day (assuming a 30 gram protein restriction). It may not be optimal to eat this amount of antioxidants at one meal. Your body will get rid of the excess, but this works for me.

Yes, it's not traditional, but I have taken the pressure off the rest of the day; I still have plenty of room and freedom. Say I have ten grams of protein at lunch, I still have 16 grams left over for dinner. I don't have to worry about eating a bunch of anything because my goals get easier for the rest of the day. It is one less thing I have to worry about or manage today. There is no rule that says you have to space out everything equally; it's impossible, trust me. A better option is making the numbers work for you, not against you.

No cooking, no dirty dishes, no nothing, just easy in every way. Go out of your way to make breakfast a win every day, rain or shine. It's a requirement in my mind. If you bomb out at breakfast, the rest of the day gets harder to make decisions on. In addition, mentally having a win at breakfast sets you up for a better outlook for the rest of the day. Commit this to memory, make breakfast easy and a win every morning. On the weekends, when I have more time Shakshuka is always a nice treat.

It's very easy to say, well I bombed at breakfast, so I just go off the diet today. Wrong. Get back on the diet at the next meal. I have fallen off the dietary wagon more times than I can count. Get back on the program at the next meal.

Sundays (or whatever day works for you)

Pick a few recipes that you like and do two things: Go grocery shopping and then cook or prepare several of everything in advance for the week. You always want to have meals on hand, ready to go in a few minutes. It's a great way to deal with urges and stress eating. My laziness was always more powerful than my cravings. Having to go out and buy food or cook a meal that takes awhile compared to something already prepared cuts down on the number of times I fell off the wagon.

Also, stop buying or keeping bad foods (the things that knock you off the diet) in the house. You don't keep booze in your house for alcoholics or heroin for addicts so don't keep foods that are bad for your kidneys in the house either.

Always be thinking "How can I make it easier?"

There is no award or trophy for making things hard on yourself, the most time consuming or most complicated diet. Go out of your way to make it easy on yourself every chance you get. I didn't say cheat on the diet, I am saying make your life easier when you can but still comply with your diet and keep track of your nutrition.

If you can, take one small step each week to make things easier (again, I didn't say cheat). Then after a few weeks, things will be super easy for you.

Desserts

I am not much of a "sweets" guy but found something odd about desserts and this diet. I added desserts to increase my calories, but the biggest impact was on my diet compliance. Pineapples with rum, pears in red wine, raspberry fool or strawberry ice cream feel pretty decadent, which is a good thing. The ice cream recipe in this book is guilt-free and will fool everyone, so indulge. In my warped mind (and maybe yours) having a dessert with dinner made it much easier for me to stick with the diet. I don't know if it is the extra calories or feeling like I was not giving up any foods, but my cravings seems to be under control when I added desserts to my evening meal.

My guess is having a dessert doesn't feel like you are on a diet. Desserts are associated with fun, not a strict diet. This made it much easier for me, for some odd reason.

I joke about this, but I actually dreamed about barbecue joints at night. That's how strong our habits can be. Eating desserts with dinner cured my barbecue joint fantasies somehow.

Yes, it takes a little extra effort, but it's worth it. Find a few desserts you like and indulge a little. Trust me, it helps on several levels. Desserts add needed calories and make you feel good, so reward yourself.

Family

Many times we will be cooking for ourselves and others. It can be hard not to eat some bad foods when your spouse or family are eating a different diet. Again, we go back to prep. If you have meals prepared in advance, then you can just heat something up and not have to make a separate meal.

The diet in this book is good for everyone, with the exception of protein content. For many meals, say two out of three for the day, you can eat the same foods. The diet is pretty tasty and you won't feel deprived if you stick with it. I promise they will like it and be healthier for it. Both of you will look and feel better.

They can try it for 90 days as well and their blood work will improve as well. My wife was amazing and ate everything I did for a few months without a single complaint (except my cooking and cleaning skills).

The rule of four

Make any meal in this book at least four or five times before you decide if you like it or not. Our taste buds acquire tastes over many years, not by tasting a teaspoon once in our life. Think about the range of foods in the world. Each culture develops their own tastes for foods based on where they live and what's available. If you make a meal in this book four times and still don't like it after the fourth time, then cross it off your list. Trying something once won't get you very far. Some of these tastes may be new to you, so give it a chance.

Attitude/perspective is everything

Be adventurous; this diet is not torture. In fact, it's the exact opposite. Getting worse each year is the real torture, getting better is not torture. It's a chance to live longer, feel better, and try new things.

I wanted to mention your perspective because of comments I get from patients saying change is hard and "how did I do it?"

Listen to me, my kidney brothers and sisters, hear me loud and clear: This kind change is wonderful, amazing, and may add years of life to your kidneys and likely you as well. It might be the start of something great for you, trust me. Don't fear change or hang on to old habits that are killing you slowly. Getting better is a great ride compared to the other ride that is all downhill.

The worst case scenario is no change, the best case is stopping your disease, the most likely case is slowing your disease dramatically and feeling and looking better.

Think about it like a bet: You have three possible outcomes:

1. You lose no money

2. You win some money

3. You win a lot of money

This diet and treatment plan is the equivalent. Everyone would take this bet! So take a chance on yourself and your future.

If you are not getting better, it's time for a change anyway. Don't let old habits or personal bias send you to an early grave. I fear the day when I can't snowboard, ride motorcycles, or keep up with my kids. I am as vain as the next person; I fear looking and acting "old." I promise you I am going down swinging. I am not going to go willingly. Who knows where I would be right now, 20+ years into an incurable disease if I hadn't been willing to change for my own good and listen to my blood tests were telling me.

It's not always easy, but it's something you don't want to miss. The people that love you don't want you to miss this ride either. We are all cheering for you, even if you don't know it.

Water

You will hear the mantra "drink more water" to improve your kidneys. Staying hydrated is certainly important, but I would caution you on the pure water approach.

We can get calories and antioxidants we need with fruit juices, teas, coffees, and so on. Let's assume you drink three glasses of iced tea and three glasses of water a day.

Teas and coffees might give you more than 100 mg of flavonoids and polyphenols per glass/cup.

Cranberry juice gives the same, plus the extra calories with no protein.

Plant-based milk adds calories with little to no protein as well.

Water is great, but a good idea is a one for one rule. For every one glass of water, you can have something else to drink. This allows you to get some needed antioxidants, calories, and variety while staying hydrated.

Focus on the real goal

Your real goal is to get through the first 90 days and see what happens. You need to stay on the plan for 90 days, come hell or high water. Find the right motivation and get with it. You will know if this diet and treatment plan can help you in 90 days. I was on strong drugs for over a year before we could determine if they worked or not. 90 days is nothing in the big picture and it's a pretty short time to see if a treatment will work for you or not.

Remember the mantra "moderation kills." Going halfway or going easy is for healthy people, not for us. Go all in for yourself and your family.

I hope these small hints help you stay on the diet and treatment plan for at least the first 90 days. All your kidneys are asking for is a 90 day vacation or sabbatical after decades of serving you and your body. Give your kidneys a 90 day break and see what happens.

CHAPTER 5

Intro to recipe section

The recipes are grouped just like you would expect: breakfast, lunch, dinner, drinks, dessert, and snacks.

I have also included a chart in the appendix showing renal acid load, protein, antioxidants, etc. of the most common fruits and veggies. This book is being printed in 8x11 format, so you have room to write on the pages.

You will have to change just about every recipe in this book a small amount to adjust for your current situation: calories per day, potassium restriction, protein restriction, personal tastes and so on. The easiest thing to do is write in the book and make notes on the recipe page and keep the book handy.

Our plan is to expand this book over time, but we want to get a basic diet and recipe guide out as soon as possible due to demand.

Estimated costs for every recipe are included. I did this for several reasons:

1. Many patients are on a fixed income, so every penny matters.

2. One of the objections to low-protein diets is cost. I will show you a single person can eat well for about $10 to $15 a day in most cases. Food costs will differ all around the world but will be pretty close for the prices in the lower 48. As you will see, it's cheaper than fast food.

3. Knowing the estimated costs may help you with planning your menu and take away any fears about costs or trying something new.

I also tried to keep special foods or special orders to a minimum. 90% of the food here can be purchased in a large local grocery store. Having lived in small towns, I recognize that specialty foods can be hard to find. If you live in the smallest of towns, you may have to drive to a larger city to shop every once in awhile. Amazon is also an option for many foods. You will have to order a few things from Amazon or other sites, but not many.

We tried it improve on my basic diet and use themes or nights: Tapas, seafood, steak, Italian, Mexican and so on. We will also note if the recipes can be frozen or keep well. For example, Gumbo Z Herbes (an old school Louisiana staple on Fridays) doesn't keep well at all. Make it on Friday night and eat over the weekend. In a few days, it will go bad.

You will see my tastes in the book for the first edition, but over time we are going to expand the book for 2020 with your input.

At the end of the recipe section, a few sample meal plans are listed. Hundreds of emails asked for everything to be calculated for them. Again, you will have to make small adjustments for your personal situation.

I will say it one more time: My personal advice is to take two or three meal plans or put together a few meal plans and then go into brain dead zombie mode. Execute the plan and don't look up again for 90 days. Thinking or complicating things is your enemy at this stage; what you need is great execution of your simple treatment and diet plan.

Here are the basic steps of the diet:

Step 1: Plan several days of meals to meet your current needs, buy the groceries, and make in advance.

Step 2: Don't look up or think for 90 days; keep executing your plan and stay on track. If you fall off the wagon, get back on at the next meal.

Step 3: Get your blood work done 90 days later.

Step 4: Watch your doctor (who said nothing could be done) be left speechless by your results and listen for the now famous line: "I don't know what your doing, but keep doing it." Take a selfie standing next to your doctor showing his/her happy, but shocked expression holding your test results and send it to me.

Step 5: Send me an email update or call me and let me know how you are doing. (Don't forget the selfie with your doctor.)

Step 6 : Party or reward time. It's important to recognize the good in life and the results of your efforts. If slowing an incurable disease is not something to celebrate, I don't know what is. Do something life affirming and fun.

(If you party first, you may forget to update me and send me a pic.)

Good Karma

You are also helping other kidney patients. Every time one of us gets good results, we educate our doctors and caregivers a little and help them get up-to-date. The average nephrologist has close to 1,000 patients. If your doctors starts seeing several of these patients get better, he or she will be more open to the next patient who wants to try it. At some point, they will suggest others try the plan. I believe this is the fastest way to get a new treatment option in the medical system. This is already happening with several nephrology programs.

Reward

Start the process over again for the next 90-day cycle and plan for an even bigger party next time. We need to keep going to get the "Goldilocks zone"; see chapter 40 in *Stopping Kidney Disease*. Once I started using rewards, my compliance got better.

Reward yourself and your significant other, who has likely been very supportive. As I said, do something life-affirming after the first successful 90 days. Something on your bucket list, take the grandkids somewhere, go on a second honeymoon, finally take the salsa dancing lessons you secretly wanted to do, sky dive, scuba dive, visit another country, hit Las Vegas or whatever. Get out there and do something fun every 90-day cycle. It's required, in my mind. It will keep you young and motivated. You can use this reward as part of your motivation. This really helped me mentally.

You and I deserve every opportunity in life and in medicine. In our case, we have to do much of it for ourselves. You need to accept responsibility for how your disease progresses, as it is largely up to you and the choices you make. We are here to help, so please use us as a resource.

I cannot say or promise what will happen when you try the diet and treatment plan for 90 days. I do know the results so far have been better than we ever imagined. The oldest patient kicking kidney ass is 88. GFR increases are being reported by multiple readers every week. The odds of something good happening for you are very high. However, hundreds of variations of kidney disease exist, along with comorbid health conditions so I want to promise something miraculous, but I can't.

However, I can say again, with complete confidence:

Every treatment plan or diet you don't try is guaranteed for fail.

I really believe we can change the outcome for kidney patients by educating each patient one at a time on how to manage this disease over the long term. I hope this book helps you more than either of us can imagine.

—*Lee*

PS: Don't forget about the selfie with your doctor and to let me know how you are doing.

Two reminders before going forward:

- You should always be under a physician's supervision and care.

- Low or very low protein diets are not safe without proper protein supplementation to ensure your protein needs are met.

Please help us improve the recipes by going to www.stoppingkidneydisease.com/recipeinput and rating recipes.

Blåbärssoppa
(Blueberry Soup)

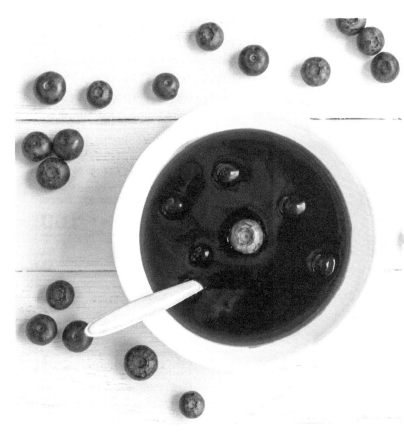

Prep Time: 5 minutes

Cook Time: 10 minutes

Serves 1

We were introduced to this recipe by Swedish friends. Our kids are involved in Nordic sports, and they asked if the kids had ever tried Blåbärssoppa (don't ask me how to say it). Needless to say, the answer was no. This soup is served in the wintertime and sometimes served before ski competitions. Blueberries are great for kidney patients due to the high antioxidants and low protein content. Two versions are included—one with vanilla coconut yogurt and the other without. Coconut yogurt is now available in most grocery stores, and Trader Joe's version is typically the lowest in price. Coconut yogurt has no protein but is high in sugar and saturated fat, so it's not perfect. However, it is a good substitute for dairy yogurt. Blueberries, on the other hand, are the perfect food for us. This recipe is simplified compared to the true Swedish version. I prefer the version without yogurt, just wild blueberries. The true Swedish version uses lemon juice, cinnamon, and cardamon. I suggest trying the plain version first, and then adjust the flavoring by adding a sweetener, lemon juice, or spices to your liking. Also, if you are trying to gain weight, use the yogurt. If you are trying to lose weight, skip the yogurt.

Ingredients:

2 cups (200 g) frozen wild blueberries

Calorie-free sweetener (such as Stevia, Splenda or Erythritol) (optional)

1 (5.3-ounce) carton (150 g) vanilla coconut yogurt (optional)

Directions:

1. Place frozen blueberries in a small saucepan and cook over medium-low heat until blueberries have released some liquid, about 5 minutes.

2. Remove from the heat, and adjust the sweetness by adding desired amount of sweetener a little at a time.

3. Let cool, and serve warm with coconut yogurt, if desired.

Notes: Add some more flavor with ¼ teaspoon ground cardamom, ¼ teaspoon ground cinnamon, and 1 teaspoon fresh lemon juice. Add these ingredients just before cooking the blueberries.

Cost Analysis:

The cost for a 4-lb bag of frozen wild blueberries runs between $9.00 (when you have a coupon or they're on sale) and $12.00. For a $12.00 4-lb. bag of blueberries, the yield is about 13 cup, so $1.84/2 cups. Coconut yogurt is a little more expensive than traditional yogurt, at around $1.50 per 5.3-oz carton. This brings the costs for the blueberry/yogurt combo to $3.90. By comparison, the cost for an egg McMuffin with hash browns is $3.79—about $0.56 more expensive, but the blueberry soup being thousand times better for you. It's not expensive to eat well. This recipe takes just a few minutes to prepare and frozen berries allow year-round consumption.

Just Blueberries

Nutrition Facts	
Serving Size	Entire Recipe
Amount Per Serving	
Calories	**100**
	Kidney Friendly % DV*
Total Fat 0.5g	1%
Saturated Fat 0g	0%
Trans Fat 0g	
Cholesterol 0mg	0%
Total Carbohydrate 30g	11%
Dietary Fiber 5g	16%
Total Sugars 20g	
Includes 0g Added Sugar	0%
Protein 1g	
Sodium 0mg	0%
Potassium 155mg	4%
Phosphorus 25mg	2%
ORAC 19240	64%
Polyphenols 445	45%
AGE	VERY LOW
PRAL	-2.1
Dietary Nitrates	VERY LOW

* The % Daily Value (DV) tells you how much a nutrient in a serving of food contributes to the daily kidney friendly diet. 2,000 calories a day is used for general nutrition advice.

With Coconut Yogurt & Splenda

Nutrition Facts	
Serving Size	Entire Recipe
Amount Per Serving	
Calories	**280**
	Kidney Friendly % DV*
Total Fat 5g	7%
Saturated Fat 4g	20%
Trans Fat 0g	
Cholesterol 0mg	0%
Total Carbohydrate 45g	16%
Dietary Fiber 5g	16%
Total Sugars 33g	
Includes 0g Added Sugar	0%
Protein 2g	
Sodium 35mg	2%
Potassium 185mg	5%
Phosphorus 35mg	3%
ORAC 19255	64%
Polyphenols 445mg	45%
AGE	VERY LOW
PRAL	-2.2
Dietary Nitrates	VERY LOW

* The % Daily Value (DV) tells you how much a nutrient in a serving of food contributes to the daily kidney friendly diet. 2,000 calories a day is used for general nutrition advice.

Creamy Breakfast Polenta with Stewed Blackberries

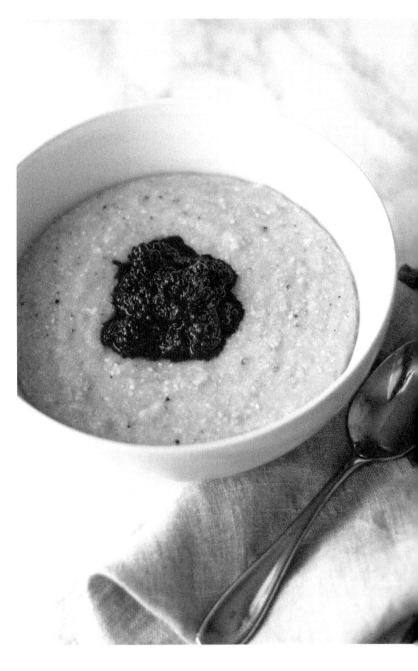

Prep Time: 5 minutes

Cook Time: 20 minutes

Serves 1

For those of us who grew up on grits or polenta, yellow corn grits are a great and very cheap option. Blackberries sounded odd to me to pair with this dish at first, but after trying it I prefer this recipe over traditional plain grits. I had to try it a few times to develop a taste for it. Remember, try each recipe four times before deciding if you like it or not. Blackberries add antioxidants and polyphenols to corn which is pretty low in nutrients.

Ingredients:

For the polenta:

½ cup + 1 tablespoon (80 g) polenta corn grits (such as Bob's Red Mill)

¼ cup (60 ml) water

¼ cup (60 ml) unenriched rice milk (such as original Rice Dream)

3 tablespoons (45 ml) coconut creamer (such as So Delicious)

Optional toppings:

¼ teaspoon (0.65 g) ground cinnamon

¼ teaspoon (1.05 g) vanilla extract

1 teaspoon (20 mg) calorie-free sweetener (such as Stevia, Splenda or Erythritol)

For the stewed blackberries:

½ cup (75 g) frozen blackberries

1 tablespoon (15 ml) water

¼ teaspoon (1.05 g) vanilla extract

¼ teaspoon (1.25 ml) fresh lemon juice

½ teaspoon (10 mg) calorie-free sweetener (such as Stevia, Splenda or Erythritol) (optional)

Directions:

1. Combine the polenta, ¼ cup water, and rice milk in a medium saucepan. Bring to a boil over medium heat; reduce heat to low and simmer, stirring frequently until polenta thickens, about 3 to 5 minutes.

2. Stir in the coconut creamer, 1 tablespoon at a time, and continue to cook, stirring until a thick porridge forms, about 5 to 7 minutes. Stir in cinnamon, vanilla extract, and sweetened, if desired.

3. While the polenta is cooking, make the blackberries. Heat the blackberries and 1 tablespoon water in a small saucepan over medium heat. When the blackberries begin to soften, use the back of a spoon to press the berries. Stir in the vanilla, lemon juice, and sweetener, if desired.

4. Continue to cook until the blackberry sauce thickens. Remove from the heat.

5. To serve, pour the polenta into a bowl, and top with the blackberry.

Note: Polenta tends to harden if not eaten right away. If you choose to make this meal ahead or make multiple servings for meal prep, pour the polenta into a large square dish and refrigerate it. To reheat, cut the polenta into squares. To make it creamy like grits or oatmeal again, add 2 to 4 tablespoons of water or plant-based milk and stir together. Heat over medium heat until creamy, and top with the stewed blackberries.

Cost Analysis:

Bob's Red Mill corn grits/polenta is available at most stores. $3.19 for a 24-ounce bag. 24 ounces will make this recipe around five to six times, so the cost for the grits is $0.63.

Frozen blackberries at Costco or Walmart come to $0.15 an ounce. A half cup of blackberries will be two to three ounces. So let's call it $0.45.

The total cost will be around $1.08 per serving.

Nutrition Facts	
Serving Size	Entire Recipe
Amount Per Serving	
Calories	**400**
	Kidney Friendly % DV*
Total Fat 3g	4%
Saturated Fat 1.5g	8%
Trans Fat 0g	
Cholesterol 0mg	0%
Total Carbohydrate 79g	29%
Dietary Fiber 9g	30%
Total Sugars 8g	
Includes 0g Added Sugar	0%
Protein 8g	
Sodium 25mg	1%
Potassium 260mg	7%
Phosphorus 95mg	8%
ORAC 15955	53%
Polyphenols 1165mg	117%
AGE	VERY LOW
PRAL	0.4
Dietary Nitrates	HIGH

* The % Daily Value (DV) tells you how much a nutrient in a serving of food contributes to the daily kidney friendly diet. 2,000 calories a day is used for general nutrition advice.

Stewed Cinnamon Apples

Prep Time: 5 minutes

Cook Time: 10 minutes

Serves 1

Apple pie for breakfast--what could be better? Ok, not exactly apple pie but pretty close. This can also be a dessert or snack of you like. Don't peel the apples. This may seem a little odd, but almost all of the antioxidants and polyphenols are in the skins.

Ingredients:

2 large apples, cored and diced

½ teaspoon (0.65 g) ground cinnamon

6 tablespoons (92 ml) water

1 tablespoon (14.2 g) non-dairy buttery spread (such as Smart balance) or real butter

1 tablespoon (6.81 g) chopped pecans (optional)

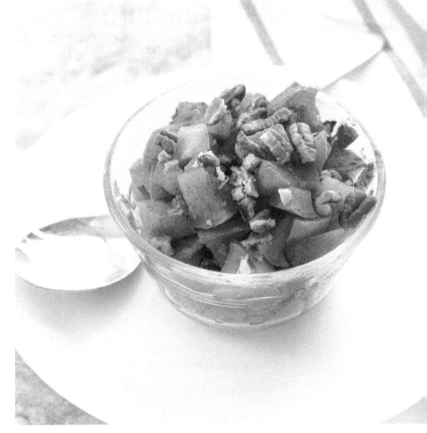

Directions:

1. Place the apples and water in a small saucepan over medium heat. Add the cinnamon and stir. Bring to a boil; cover, reduce heat to low and simmer 6 to 8 minutes.

2. Uncover, and cook, stirring frequently, until the apples are soft and the water evaporates. Add 1 tablespoon of water, if needed, if the apples appear to be too dry. Stir in the buttery spread.

3. To serve, spoon the apples into a serving bowl and top with chopped pecans.

Cost Analysis:

Apples are pretty cheap per pound depending on what kind you buy. This recipe will cost less than $2.00 even if you buy some of the most expensive apples. As a rule, darker red is better from an antioxidant point of view, but go with whatever looks best in the store.

Nutrition Facts

Serving Size	Entire Recipe

Amount Per Serving

Calories	395

	Kidney Friendly % DV*
Total Fat 17g	22%
Saturated Fat 8g	39%
Trans Fat 0g	
Cholesterol 30mg	10%
Total Carbohydrate 67g	24%
Dietary Fiber 12g	41%
Total Sugars 49g	
Includes 0g Added Sugar	0%
Protein 2g	
Sodium 5mg	0%
Potassium 540mg	15%
Phosphorus 75mg	6%
ORAC 16470	55%
Polyphenols 1095mg	109%
AGE	MEDIUM
PRAL	-9.1
Dietary Nitrates	LOW

* The % Daily Value (DV) tells you how much a nutrient in a serving of food contributes to the daily kidney friendly diet. 2,000 calories a day is used for general nutrition advice.

Huevo Ranchero
(Omelet with Pepper & Onion Hash)

Prep Time: 10 minutes

Cook Time: 10 minutes

Serves 1

Egg whites are much lower in acid than the egg with the yolk. Egg whites are also easy to find these days or you can just separate at home. You have to watch protein the rest of the day if you start the day with an egg-based recipe. The positives are it may help with cravings, and egg whites supply all of the essential amino acids. You can do it two ways with a red pepper hash or Shakshuka (my favorite), but many of us grew up on hash so we are providing both.

Ingredients:

For the Omelet:

2 egg whites

1 tablespoon (15 ml) unenriched rice milk (such as original Rice Dream)

2 teaspoons (9.15 g) olive or avocado oil, divided

¼ teaspoon (1.42 g) salt

¼ teaspoon (0.57 g) freshly ground black pepper

For the Hash:

1 teaspoon (4.57 g) olive or avocado oil

3 tablespoons (30 g) diced red onion

½ cup (90 g) diced red bell pepper

⅛ teaspoon (0.25 g) garlic powder

Pinch of freshly ground black pepper

2 tablespoons (6 g) chopped fresh cilantro

Directions:

1. Whisk together the egg, rice milk, 1 teaspoon oil, salt, and pepper. Heat the remaining 1 teaspoon oil in a small nonstick skillet over medium heat Once the skillet is hot, pour in the egg mixture and carefully swirl the egg around to coat the bottom of the pan. Reduce the heat to medium-low, and cover the pan with a lid.

2. Allow the egg to cook for 30 to 45 seconds, or until set. Once the edges of the eggs are cooked and the egg feels fairly firm underneath, carefully flip over the egg using a small flexible non-stick spatula. Allow the egg to cook on the other side until it is fully cooked and no longer runny. Remove the omelet from the skillet, and keep warm.

3. Wipe out the skillet and add 1 teaspoon oil. Place over medium heat and add the onion. Sauté for about 2 minutes or until softened. Add the bell pepper and sauté 2 to 3 minutes or until the peppers are softened. Stir in the garlic powder and a pinch of salt and pepper. Remove the hash from the heat, and stir in the chopped cilantro.

4. To serve, place the omelet on a plate and top with the hash.

Note: This is an excellent recipe to scale up to enjoy throughout the week. You can make one large egg omelet and cut into individual servings. Or, hard-boil a few eggs and chop one up to stir into the hash.

Cost Analysis:

If we assume $1.50 for the red pepper, $0.15 per ounce for commercial egg whites, and $0.50 for the rice and coconut cramer, we still come in less than $2.50 for this recipe.

Nutrition Facts	
Serving Size	220g
Amount Per Serving	
Calories	**210**
	Kidney Friendly % DV*
Total Fat 14g	**18%**
Saturated Fat 2g	**10%**
Trans Fat 0g	
Cholesterol 0mg	**0%**
Total Carbohydrate 12g	**4%**
Dietary Fiber 3g	**10%**
Total Sugars 6g	
Includes 0g Added Sugar	**0%**
Protein 13g	
Sodium 760mg	35%
Potassium 490mg	14%
Phosphorus 60mg	5%
ORAC 1870	6%
Polyphenols 210mg	21%
AGE	LOW
PRAL	-3.2
Dietary Nitrates	LOW

* The % Daily Value (DV) tells you how much a nutrient in a serving of food contributes to the daily kidney friendly diet. 2,000 calories a day is used for general nutrition advice.

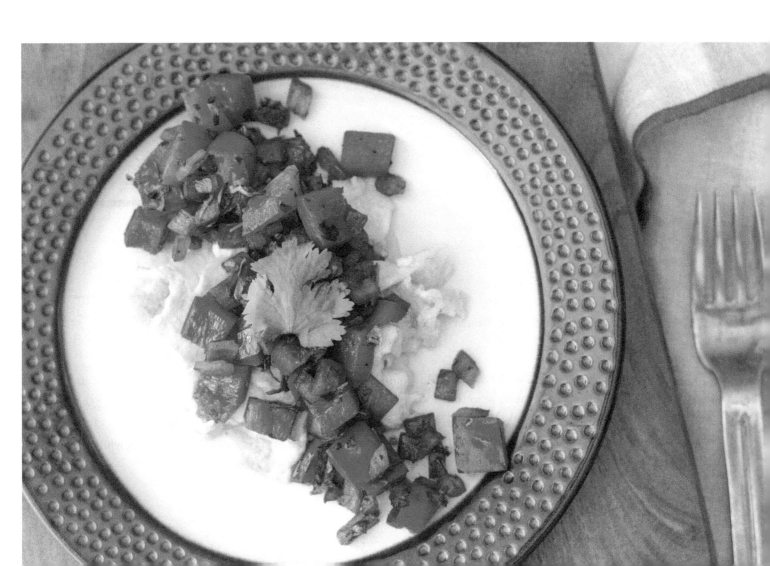

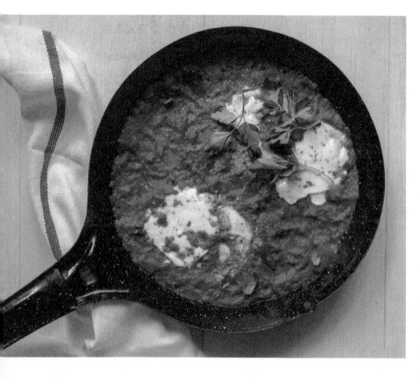

Shakshuka

Prep Time: 10 minutes

Cook Time: 10 minutes

Serves 1

For the record, Shakshuka is the bomb. The original version is tomato based. This version only has one tomato to limit potassium. A spicy, warm dish topped with two egg whites can go a long way to satisfy my cravings. You can make it as spicy or as mild as you like. I think the best way is to take half of the non egg ingredients and process in a blender and leave the other half of the mixture in larger diced pieces for some texture and crunch. It can turn a little soupy if you put 100% in the blender. You can also make the "sauce" in advance and freeze to have on hand. Microwave the sauce on low or thaw in a skillet.

Ingredients:

2 teaspoons (9.15 g) olive oil

½ red bell pepper, seeded and diced (¾ cup; 135 g)

½ tomato, chopped (⅓ cup; 65 g)

1 carrot, peeled and diced (¼ cup; 40 g)

¼ cup (40 g) chopped onion

½ teaspoon (0.5 g) ground cumin

¼ teaspoon (0.25 g) paprika

¼ teaspoon (0.25 g) garlic powder

¼ teaspoon (1.42 g) salt

¼ teaspoon (0.57 g) pepper

¼ cup (60 ml) water

2 egg whites

Chopped fresh parsley or cilantro (optional)

Nutrition Facts	
Serving Size	Entire Recipe
Amount Per Serving	
Calories	**200**
	Kidney Friendly % DV*
Total Fat 10g	13%
Saturated Fat 1.5g	8%
Trans Fat 0g	
Cholesterol 0mg	0%
Total Carbohydrate 20g	7%
Dietary Fiber 6g	19%
Total Sugars 11g	
Includes 0g Added Sugar	0%
Protein 11g	
Sodium 695mg	32%
Potassium 770mg	22%
Phosphorus 90mg	8%
ORAC 1485	5%
Polyphenols 105mg	10%
AGE	VERY LOW
PRAL	-9.1
Dietary Nitrates	LOW

* The % Daily Value (DV) tells you how much a nutrient in a serving of food contributes to the daily kidney friendly diet. 2,000 calories a day is used for general nutrition advice.

Directions:

1. Heat the oil in a skillet over medium-high heat, and sauté the bell pepper, tomato, carrot, onion, and seasonings 8 minutes or until tender. Process with an immersion blender (or use a stand blender), leaving some chunks if desired.

2. Create 2 wells in the sauce and add the egg whites. Cover and cook 3 minutes or until egg whites are firm. Sprinkle with parsley or cilantro, if desired.

Cost Analysis:

Shakshuka is roughly the same cost as the Ranchero coming in under $2.50.

Fruit bowl

Prep Time: 5 minutes

Serves 1

This dish is simple, fast, easy to measure, cheap, and super healthy.

Ingredients:

2 cups (200 g) (or a combination of) blackberries, blueberries, raspberries, or strawberries

1 (5.3-ounce)(150 g) carton vanilla coconut yogurt (optional)

Directions:

Combine desired mixture of berries in a serving bowl. Serve with coconut yogurt, if desired.

Cost Analysis:

The cost for strawberries, cultivated blueberries, and blackberries will be around $1.00 per cup. Raspberries will be closer to $2.50 a cup. This recipe will cost $2.00 to $5.00 depending on the fruit used and an additional $1.60 for the coconut yogurt.

Nutrition Facts	
Serving Size	Entire Recipe
Amount Per Serving	
Calories	**165**
	Kidney Friendly % DV*
Total Fat 6g	7%
Saturated Fat 2g	12%
Trans Fat 0g	
Cholesterol 0mg	0%
Total Carbohydrate 35g	13%
Dietary Fiber 11g	35%
Total Sugars 22g	
Includes 0g Added Sugar	0%
Protein 3g	
Sodium 15mg	1%
Potassium 355mg	10%
Phosphorus 100mg	8%
ORAC 38455	128%
Polyphenols 1140mg	114%
AGE	VERY LOW
PRAL	-6.6
Dietary Nitrates	HIGH

* The % Daily Value (DV) tells you how much a nutrient in a serving of food contributes to the daily kidney friendly diet. 2,000 calories a day is used for general nutrition advice.

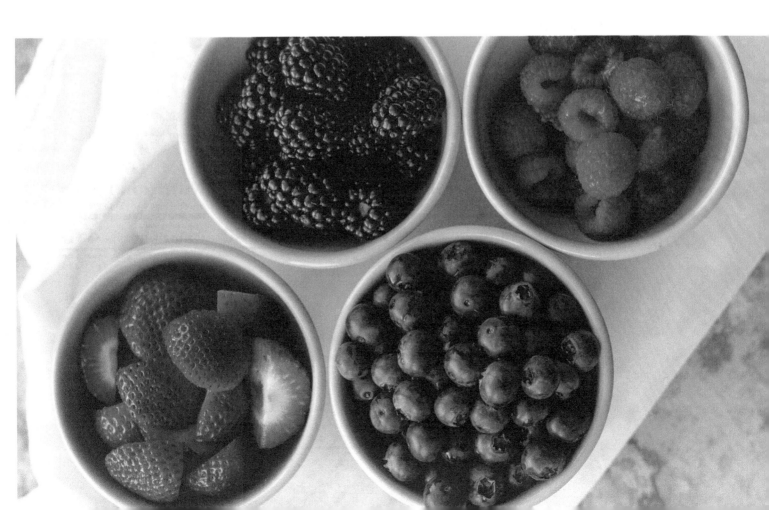

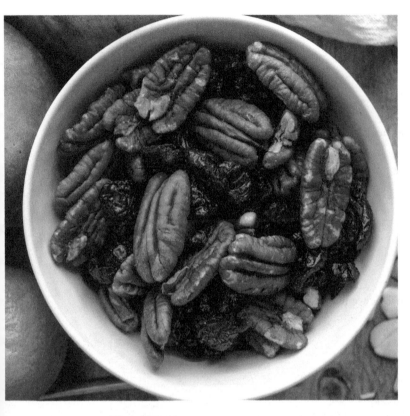

Pecan and Fruit Bowls

Prep Time: 5 minutes

Serves 1

This has become my go-to breakfast. I used to use toasted pecans but got lazy. I just use pecans right out of the bag. This is a very healthy breakfast with good calories, and you can eat it on the run or as a meal. This one of those meals you cannot have often enough. If you are on a car trip, it's a great recipe to throw in a ziplock bag. Choose whatever fruit is in season.

Ingredients:

⅓ cup (40 g) reduced-sugar dried cranberries (such as Craisins)

¼ cup (30 g) pecan halves

1 apple, pear, or small tangerine (halo or cutie)

Directions:

Combine the cranberries, pecan halves, and apple, pear, or tangerine in a serving bowl or eat separately.

Breakfast twist: Make this a cereal-inspired breakfast: Chop the pecans and apple or pear, sprinkle with a pinch of ground cinnamon, and top with a milk substitute. This adds calories and may satisfy a craving is you have been having cereal for breakfast for years.

Cost Analysis:

Reduced-sugar dried cranberries will cost $0.35 to $0.40. Pecans will add another $0.35 to $0.40, and the fruit cost will vary, but will almost always be less than $0.75. This recipe will run between $1.40 and $1.75 in most cases.

Apple

Nutrition Facts	
Serving Size	Entire Recipe
Amount Per Serving	
Calories	**390**
	Kidney Friendly % DV*
Total Fat 22g	**28%**
Saturated Fat 2g	**9%**
Trans Fat 0g	
Cholesterol 0mg	**0%**
Total Carbohydrate 57g	**21%**
Dietary Fiber 17g	**56%**
Total Sugars 32g	
Includes 6g Added Sugar	**12%**
Protein 3g	
Sodium 0mg	0%
Potassium 310mg	9%
Phosphorus 105mg	8%
ORAC 13835	46%
Polyphenols 830mg	83%
AGE	VERY LOW
PRAL	-2.7
Dietary Nitrates	HIGH

* The % Daily Value (DV) tells you how much a nutrient in a serving of food contributes to the daily kidney friendly diet. 2,000 calories a day is used for general nutrition advice.

Clementine

Nutrition Facts	
Serving Size	145g
Amount Per Serving	
Calories	**340**
	Kidney Friendly % DV*
Total Fat 22g	**28%**
Saturated Fat 2g	**9%**
Trans Fat 0g	
Cholesterol 0mg	**0%**
Total Carbohydrate 44g	**16%**
Dietary Fiber 14g	**47%**
Total Sugars 22g	
Includes 6g Added Sugar	**12%**
Protein 3g	
Sodium 0mg	0%
Potassium 270mg	8%
Phosphorus 100mg	8%
ORAC 10595	35%
Polyphenols 720mg	72%
AGE	VERY LOW
PRAL	-2
Dietary Nitrates	HIGH

* The % Daily Value (DV) tells you how much a nutrient in a serving of food contributes to the daily kidney friendly diet. 2,000 calories a day is used for general nutrition advice.

Pear

Nutrition Facts	
Serving Size	Entire Recipe
Amount Per Serving	
Calories	**410**
	Kidney Friendly % DV*
Total Fat 22g	**28%**
Saturated Fat 2g	**9%**
Trans Fat 0g	
Cholesterol 0mg	**0%**
Total Carbohydrate 63g	**23%**
Dietary Fiber 18g	**61%**
Total Sugars 33g	
Includes 6g Added Sugar	**12%**
Protein 3g	
Sodium 0mg	0%
Potassium 350mg	10%
Phosphorus 105mg	9%
ORAC 12950	43%
Polyphenols 705mg	70%
AGE	VERY LOW
PRAL	-3.8
Dietary Nitrates	HIGH

* The % Daily Value (DV) tells you how much a nutrient in a serving of food contributes to the daily kidney friendly diet. 2,000 calories a day is used for general nutrition advice.

Green Pineapple Smoothie

Prep Time: 10 minutes

Serves 2

There are an unlimited amount of smoothie recipes available. Be careful with potassium, acid, and protein load. Pineapple is anti-inflammatory and arugula and cilantro and great for your heart and kidneys.

Ingredients:

1 ½ cups (367.5 g) frozen pineapple chunks

2 cups (40 g) baby arugula

⅓ cup (15 g) chopped fresh cilantro

¾ cup (177 ml) unenriched rice milk (such as original Rice Dream)

2 tablespoons (30 ml) coconut creamer (such as So Delicious)

Directions:

Combine pineapple, arugula, cilantro, rice milk, and coconut creamer, if desired, in a blender. Pulse until mixture is smooth. Pour into serving glasses, and serve immediately.

Cost Analysis:

The cost with all ingredients will run around $2.30 to $2.50 per recipe.

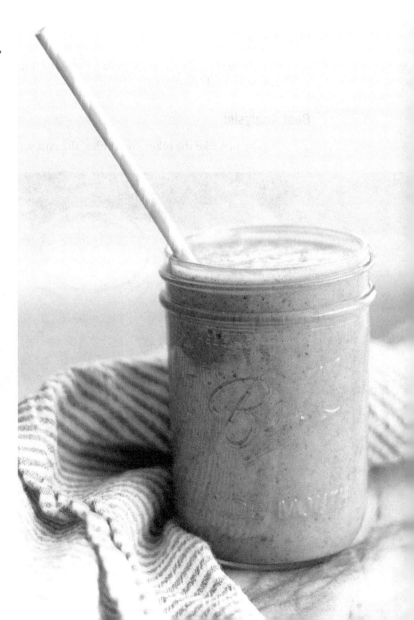

Nutrition Facts

Serving Size	1/2 Recipe

Amount Per Serving

Calories	155

	Kidney Friendly % DV*
Total Fat 2g	2%
Saturated Fat 0.5g	3%
Trans Fat 0g	
Cholesterol 0mg	0%
Total Carbohydrate 34g	12%
Dietary Fiber 3g	12%
Total Sugars 23g	
Includes 0g Added Sugar	0%
Protein 2g	
Sodium 50mg	2%
Potassium 340mg	10%
Phosphorus 50mg	4%
ORAC 1800	6%
Polyphenols 310mg	31%
AGE	VERY LOW
PRAL	-6.2
Dietary Nitrates	MEDIUM

* The % Daily Value (DV) tells you how much a nutrient in a serving of food contributes to the daily kidney friendly diet. 2,000 calories a day is used for general nutrition advice.

Basic Fruit Smoothie

Prep Time: 10 minutes

Serves 1

Any low potassium fruit will do--strawberries, blueberries, raspberries, blackberries apples, pears and so on. Blackberries and raspberries have small seeds that some will not like in their smoothie. Adding a tangerine helps the flavor and increases the nutritional value.

Ingredients:

2 cups (288 g) strawberries

1 small tangerine (halo or cutie)

3 tablespoons (45 ml) unenriched rice milk (such as original Rice Dream)

1 tablespoon (15 ml) coconut creamer (such as So Delicious)

Water or ice cubes, as needed

Directions:

Combine ingredients in a blender. Pulse until mixture is smooth, adding water or ice cubes as needed to reach desired consistency.

Cost Analysis:

Again, just like the other smoothies, the cost will run between $2.00 to $2.50 in most cases.

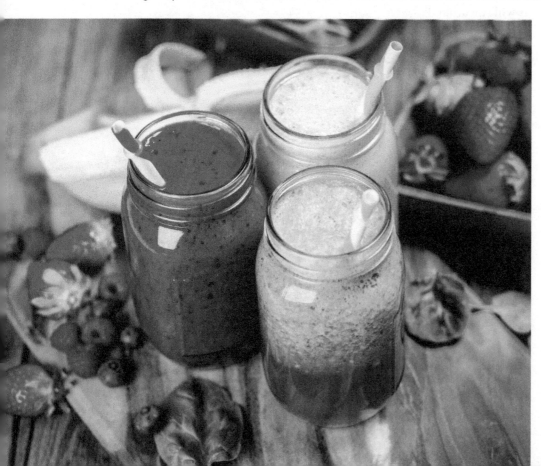

Nutrition Facts		
Serving Size		Entire Recipe
Amount Per Serving		
Calories		**160**
		Kidney Friendly % DV*
Total Fat 2g		3%
Saturated Fat 0.5g		2%
Trans Fat 0g		
Cholesterol 0mg		0%
Total Carbohydrate 35g		13%
Dietary Fiber 7g		23%
Total Sugars 22g		
Includes 0g Added Sugar		0%
Protein 3g		
Sodium 25mg		1%
Potassium 580mg		17%
Phosphorus 95mg		8%
ORAC 13950		47%
Polyphenols 1040mg		104%
AGE		VERY LOW
PRAL		-9.6
Dietary Nitrates		HIGH

* The % Daily Value (DV) tells you how much a nutrient in a serving of food contributes to the daily kidney friendly diet. 2,000 calories a day is used for general nutrition advice.

Beet Salad with Candied or Spiced Pecans

Prep Time: 20 minutes

Cook Time: 20 minutes

Serves 1

This has become my go-to lunch. It's about as close to a perfect meal for a kidney patient as you can get. Heart healthy and high antioxidant pecans, arugula, and beets for nitric oxide increases blood flow. High antioxidant and high fiber cranberries also pack a lot of nutrition punch. Use canned beets to reduce potassium, and read the labels. Many have added corn syrup (do not use these.) Amazon has the 365 Everyday Value brand with no salt and no corn syrup. You can't have this salad too much. The pecans add crunch and cranberries add a chewy factor to make it a very satisfying meal. This is a great salad to double or triple in size! Simply prepare all ingredients and leave the dressing and pecans on the side until you are ready to serve. To save time, buy pre-washed arugula in bags or clamshells.

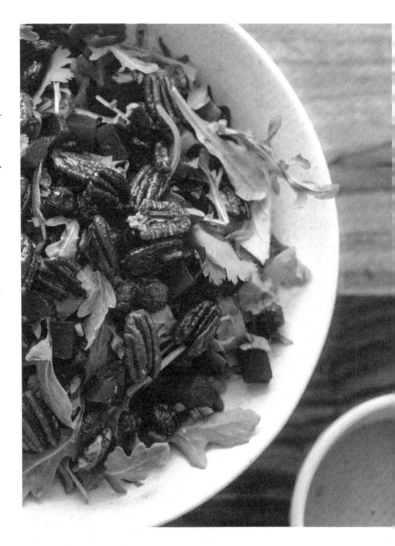

Ingredients:

For the candied pecans:

¼ cup (30 g) pecan halves

1 teaspoon (4.57 g) olive, canola, or avocado oil

1 teaspoon (20 mg) calorie-free sweetener (such as Splenda, granulated Stevia, or Erythritol)

For the spiced pecans:

¼ cup (30 g) pecan halves

1 teaspoon (4.57 g) olive, canola, or avocado oil

Pinch of cayenne pepper or ½ teaspoon curry powder

For the dressing:

2 tablespoons (27.44 g) olive oil

1 teaspoon (5.19 g) Dijon mustard

¼ teaspoon (0.5 g) garlic powder

1½ teaspoons (8 g) balsamic vinegar

Pinch of salt and pepper

For the salad:

1 cup (200 g) no-salt-added (and no corn syrup) canned beet slices

2 cups (40 g) arugula

1 cup (20 g) watercress (or use more arugula)

1 cup (16 g) chopped fresh cilantro

½ cup (60 g) reduced-sugar dried cranberries (such as Craisins)

Directions:

1. To make candied pecans, preheat the oven to 325°F. Toss the pecans in oil in a small bowl. Add half of the sugar substitute and toss to combine. Transfer to a parchment paper-rimmed baking sheet and spread in one layer. Bake for 10 minutes; stir and sprinkle the remaining sugar substitute on top of the pecans. Return to oven and bake 5 to 10 minutes longer, or until pecans are crisp.

2. To make spiced pecans, preheat the oven to 325°F. Toss the pecans in oil in a small bowl. Add the cayenne pepper or curry powder and toss to combine. Transfer to a parchment paper-rimmed baking sheet and spread in one layer. Bake for about 3 to 6 minutes or until pecans are toasted. Pecans burn easily so keep an eye on them, checking frequently.

3. To make the dressing, combine all of the dressing ingredients in a blender or in a jar and shake to combine. Season with salt and pepper to taste.

4. For the salad, drain the beets and rinse with water. Repeat the process one more time. Place the beets on paper towels to drain. Dice the beets.

5. If the arugula is large, chop if desired. Toss the arugula, watercress, and cilantro together in a serving bowl. Add the beets and dried cranberries.

6. Drizzle the salad with dressing, and toss gently to combine. Top with candied or spiced pecans.

Make Ahead: Keep the salad, pecans, and dressing separate until ready to serve.

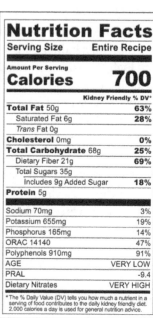

Nutrition Facts	
Serving Size	Entire Recipe
Amount Per Serving	
Calories	**700**
	Kidney Friendly % DV*
Total Fat 50g	63%
Saturated Fat 6g	28%
Trans Fat 0g	
Cholesterol 0mg	0%
Total Carbohydrate 68g	25%
Dietary Fiber 21g	69%
Total Sugars 35g	
Includes 9g Added Sugar	18%
Protein 5g	
Sodium 70mg	3%
Potassium 655mg	19%
Phosphorus 165mg	14%
ORAC 14140	47%
Polyphenols 910mg	91%
AGE	VERY LOW
PRAL	-9.4
Dietary Nitrates	VERY HIGH

* The % Daily Value (DV) tells you how much a nutrient in a serving of food contributes to the daily kidney friendly diet. 2,000 calories a day is used for general nutrition advice.

Cost Analysis:

The estimated cost is between $2.50 and $3.00 per meal.

Corn and Chile Soup with Smoky Collard Greens

Prep Time: 25 minutes

Cook Time: 30 minutes (including Smoky Collard Greens recipe)

Serves 3

I have tried to make New Mexican green chile stew for some time. However, the potassium is always too high and nutrition is on the low side. This version uses corn to replace potatoes and greens to add to the nutrition and reduce the acid load. My wife likes the greens in the soup, but i prefer the greens as a side dish with the soup. Chop the greens well if you add them to the soup. Collard greens should be on your list of foods you try to eat every week.

Ingredients:

1 tablespoon (13.63 g) olive oil

¾ cup (115 g) diced yellow onions

2 cloves garlic, minced

3 cups (396 g) frozen cauliflower florets, thawed

2 cups (350 g) frozen corn kernels, thawed

2 cups (700 ml) salt-free vegetable broth

1½ to 2 tablespoons (22.68 g) diced green chiles (such as Ortega)

2 cups (700 ml) non-dairy milk

Smoky Collard Greens (recipe follows)

Smoked paprika, for garnish

Fresh cilantro, for garnish

Directions:

1. Heat the oil in a saucepan over medium heat. Add onion and sauté for 3 to 4 minutes or until onion is soft and begins to become translucent. Stir in the garlic.

2. Add the cauliflower, 1 ½ cups of the corn kernels, and the broth. Bring to a boil; cover, reduce heat and simmer 7 to 10 minutes, or until the cauliflower is tender.

3. Stir in the chiles and non-dairy milk. Transfer half of the soup to a blender and puree until smooth. Return the pureed soup to the remaining soup in the saucepan.

4. Stir in remaining ½ cup corn and simmer for 3 to 5 minutes longer. Divide soup evenly between serving bowls and top with Smoky Collard Greens. Garnish with smoked paprika and cilantro, if desired.

Cost Analysis:

The combination of soup and collard greens came to $2.75 per serving.

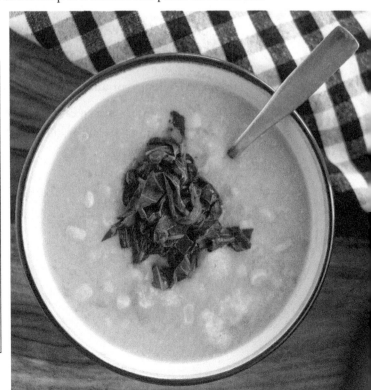

Nutrition Facts		
Serving Size		1/3 Recipe
Amount Per Serving		
Calories		**310**
		Kidney Friendly % DV*
Total Fat 10g		13%
Saturated Fat 1g		4%
Trans Fat 0g		
Cholesterol 0mg		0%
Total Carbohydrate 58g		21%
Dietary Fiber 8g		27%
Total Sugars 18g		
Includes 0g Added Sugar		0%
Protein 7g		
Sodium 160mg		7%
Potassium 490mg		14%
Phosphorus 170mg		14%
ORAC 28550		95%
Polyphenols 625mg		62%
AGE		LOW
PRAL		-4
Dietary Nitrates		MEDIUM

* The % Daily Value (DV) tells you how much a nutrient in a serving of food contributes to the daily kidney friendly diet. 2,000 calories a day is used for general nutrition advice.

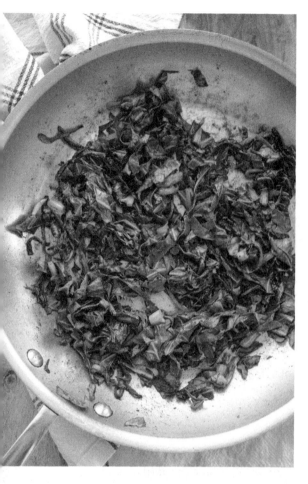

Smoky Collard Greens

Prep Time: 10 minutes

Cook Time: 15 minutes

Serves 3

Collard greens are a staple in the Deep South. They are one of the lowest potassium cruciferous veggies. Collards and other cruciferous veggies contain glucosinolates, which reportedly reduce the risk of breast, colon, and lung cancers. Collards are a great source of vitamin K , vitamin A, are high in fiber, and have a decent amount of antioxidants. They are also cheap and easy to find.

Ingredients:

1½ tablespoons (20.45 g) olive oil

½ cup (75 g) thinly sliced red onions (optional)

4 cloves garlic, sliced

5 cups (180 g) thinly sliced collard greens

½ teaspoon (0.75 g) smoked paprika

1 to 2 tablespoons (28.3 g) salt-free vegetable broth or water, as needed

Directions:

1. Heat olive oil in a heavy pot or skillet over medium high heat. Add the red onion and sauté 2 to 3 minutes, or until onions soften.

2. Add garlic and stir constantly until fragrant (but not burned).

3. Add the collard greens and smoked paprika; sauté over medium heat until collards soften. Add broth or water 1 tablespoon at a time, if needed, to prevent the collards from burning. Continue sautéing for about 3 minutes, or until the collards are tender.

Make Ahead: This recipe can easily be made ahead and stored in the refrigerator. Microwave in 30-second intervals until warmed through.

Cost Analysis:

A bunch of collard greens at my local store is under $1.00. Garlic is also cheap.

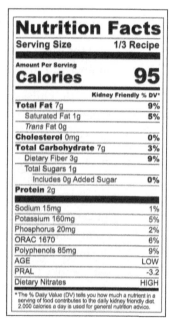

Nutrition Facts		
Serving Size		1/3 Recipe
Amount Per Serving		
Calories		**95**
		Kidney Friendly % DV*
Total Fat 7g		9%
Saturated Fat 1g		5%
Trans Fat 0g		
Cholesterol 0mg		0%
Total Carbohydrate 7g		3%
Dietary Fiber 3g		9%
Total Sugars 1g		
Includes 0g Added Sugar		0%
Protein 2g		
Sodium 15mg		1%
Potassium 160mg		5%
Phosphorus 20mg		2%
ORAC 1670		6%
Polyphenols 85mg		9%
AGE		LOW
PRAL		-3.2
Dietary Nitrates		HIGH

* The % Daily Value (DV) tells you how much a nutrient in a serving of food contributes to the daily kidney friendly diet. 2,000 calories a day is used for general nutrition advice.

Tostada Salad

Prep Time: 15 minutes

Cook Time: 25 minutes

Serves 1

This is a common salad at Mexican restaurants. Don't toss anything with the crumbled tostada until you are ready to eat. It will get soggy and lose some crunch if you let it sit too long. Tostadas are not a health food by any standard, but everything else in the salad is. If you do add the corn to the salad, it'll add 5 grams of protein.

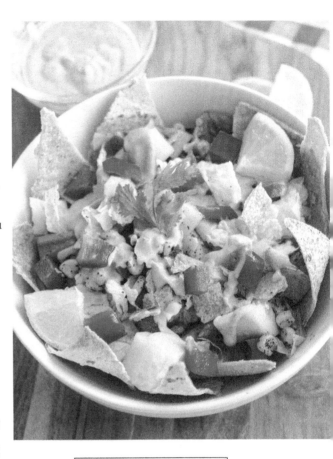

Ingredients:

For the dressing:

1½ teaspoons (6.86 g) olive oil

1 tablespoon (15 g) fresh lime juice

1 clove garlic, minced

2 tablespoons (2 g) chopped fresh cilantro

Water, as needed

For the salad:

½ cup (90 g) frozen corn kernels (optional)

1 teaspoon (4.57 g) olive oil

¼ teaspoon (0.25 g) chili powder

⅛ teaspoon (0.12 g) garlic powder

1½ cups (115 g) chopped iceberg or romaine lettuce

½ cup (66.5 g) chopped cucumber

¼ cup (45 g) chopped red bell pepper

2 corn tostadas

Directions:

1. To make the dressing, combine all of the dressing ingredients in a blender and process until smooth, adding water as needed to reach desired consistency.

2. Preheat the oven to 400°F. Toss the frozen corn with 1 teaspoon olive oil on baking sheet. Bake for 5 minutes or until corn is thawed. Stir in chili powder and garlic powder and return to the oven. Bake 10 minutes or until corn is roasted. Set aside.

3. To assemble the salad, toss together the lettuce, cucumber, bell pepper, and roasted corn in a serving bowl. Coarsely chop or crumble the tostadas; add half to the salad and arrange the remaining around the edges. Drizzle with dressing, and serve.

Make Ahead: Store the salad, dressing, and crumbled tostadas separate and then toss together once ready to eat.

Cost Analysis:

You can buy corn tostadas in any grocery store these days. The estimated cost for this meal is around $2.00

Nutrition Facts		
Serving Size		Entire Recipe
Amount Per Serving		
Calories		**360**
		Kidney Friendly % DV*
Total Fat 19g		24%
Saturated Fat 5g		24%
Trans Fat 0g		
Cholesterol 0mg		0%
Total Carbohydrate 47g		17%
Dietary Fiber 8g		25%
Total Sugars 16g		
Includes 0g Added Sugar		0%
Protein 7g		
Sodium 25mg		1%
Potassium 705mg		20%
Phosphorus 17mg		15%
ORAC 12460		42%
Polyphenols 625mg		63%
AGE		LOW
PRAL		-8.9
Dietary Nitrates		MEDIUM

* The % Daily Value (DV) tells you how much a nutrient in a serving of food contributes to the daily kidney friendly diet. 2,000 calories a day is used for general nutrition advice.

Pumpkin Chili

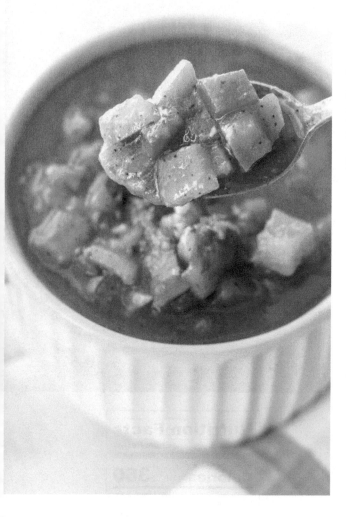

Prep Time: 20 minutes

Cook Time: 25 minutes

Serves 2

Pumpkins are actually really good for us, and this is a great fall recipe. Pumpkin-based chili may sound odd at first, but give it a try.

Ingredients:

1½ tablespoons (20.45 g) olive oil

½ cup (75 g) diced onion

¼ cup (45 g) diced green bell pepper

½ cup (90 g) diced red bell pepper

¾ cup (190 g) diced eggplant

1 cup (150 g) diced zucchini

3 cloves garlic, minced

1 teaspoon (2.71 g) chili powder

½ teaspoon (0.5 g) dried oregano

¼ teaspoon (0.25 g) ground coriander

½ teaspoon (0.5 g) ground cumin

2¼ cups (509 ml) salt-free vegetable broth

½ cup (115 g) pumpkin puree

2 tablespoons (2 g) chopped fresh cilantro

Directions:

1. Heat the oil in a Dutch oven over medium heat. Add the onion, green pepper and red peppers. Once the onion begins to soften, add the eggplant and zucchini.

2. When the eggplant absorbs the oil, add the garlic and stir until fragrant. Stir in chili powder, oregano, coriander, and cumin and stir to combine.

3. Stir in the vegetable broth and the pumpkin puree. Bring to a boil; cover, reduce heat and simmer over medium-low heat for about 15 minutes. Stir in additional vegetable broth or water if needed if the liquid reduces too much. Cook until the chili reaches desired thickness, stir in the cilantro before serving.

Make Ahead: This recipe is ideal for prepping ahead. Store in an airtight container and microwave in 30-second intervals until warmed through.

Cost Analysis:

Make sure you buy the pure canned pumpkin instead of seasoned pumpkin pie filling. A can of pumpkin costs around $2.00, which will last you awhile. The total cost with the other added veggies will be around $2.50 per serving.

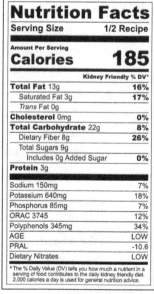

Nutrition Facts		
Serving Size		1/2 Recipe
Amount Per Serving		
Calories		**185**
		Kidney Friendly % DV*
Total Fat 13g		16%
Saturated Fat 3g		17%
Trans Fat 0g		
Cholesterol 0mg		0%
Total Carbohydrate 22g		8%
Dietary Fiber 8g		26%
Total Sugars 9g		
Includes 0g Added Sugar		0%
Protein 3g		
Sodium 150mg		7%
Potassium 640mg		18%
Phosphorus 85mg		7%
ORAC 3745		12%
Polyphenols 345mg		34%
AGE		LOW
PRAL		-10.6
Dietary Nitrates		LOW

* The % Daily Value (DV) tells you how much a nutrient in a serving of food contributes to the daily kidney friendly diet. 2,000 calories a day is used for general nutrition advice.

Baked Sweet Potato with Side Salad
Choice of Curry-Ginger Vinaigrette or Lemon-Herb Vinaigrette

Prep Time: 20 minutes

Cook Time: 25 minutes

Serves 1

This was my go-to lunch for quite a while. It's a very simple recipe for a baked sweet potato and salad, but what makes it special is the vinaigrettes. It's easy to make and travels well if you are taking to work. I think curry powder is one of the best to pair with sweet potatoes. You can also use butter or Smart balance if you like.

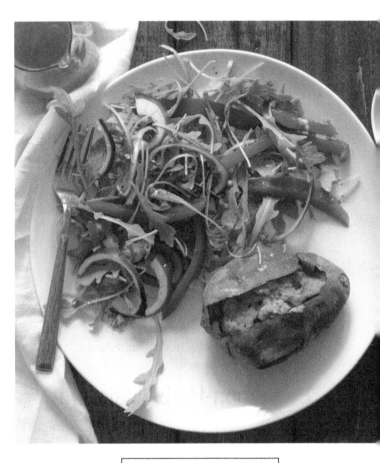

Ingredients:

For the sweet potato:

1 (4-ounce) (115 g) sweet potato

1 tablespoon spreadable non-dairy butter (such as Smart Balance)

½ teaspoon Italian seasoning

¼ teaspoon salt

¼ teaspoon pepper

1 clove garlic, minced

For the salad:

½ red bell pepper

3 cups (60 g) baby arugula

¼ red onion, thinly sliced

2 tablespoons Curry-Ginger Vinaigrette or Lemon-Herb Vinaigrette (recipes follow)

Nutrition Facts	
Serving Size	Entire Recipe
Amount Per Serving	
Calories	**180**
	Kidney Friendly % DV*
Total Fat 5g	6%
Saturated Fat 0g	0%
Trans Fat 0g	
Cholesterol 0mg	0%
Total Carbohydrate 31g	12%
Dietary Fiber 6g	19%
Total Sugars 11g	
Includes 0g Added Sugar	0%
Protein 4g	
Sodium 705mg	32%
Potassium 665mg	19%
Phosphorus 95mg	8%
ORAC 3328	11%
Polyphenols 330mg	33%
AGE	VERY LOW
PRAL	-11.8
Dietary Nitrates	MEDIUM

* The % Daily Value (DV) tells you how much a nutrient in a serving of food contributes to the daily kidney friendly diet. 2,000 calories a day is used for general nutrition advice.

Directions:

1. Preheat the oven to 400°F. Bake the sweet potato 30 minutes or until tender. Remove from the oven, split, and top with butter, seasoning, salt, pepper, and garlic. keep warm.

2. Increase the oven temperature to broil. Broil the pepper until blistered. Remove to a bowl and cover to allow the steam to soften. Remove the skin, stems, and seeds, and thinly slice.

3. To serve, combine the bell pepper, arugula, and red onion. Drizzle with desired dressing and serve with baked sweet potato (remove the skin).

Curry-Ginger Vinaigrette

Makes about ⅓ cup

Ingredients:

1 clove garlic, minced

1 teaspoon (2 g) minced fresh ginger

½ tablespoon (1.5 g) curry powder

1 tablespoon (14.3 g) apple cider vinegar

¼ teaspoon (1.42 g) salt

¼ teaspoon (0.57 g) pepper

¼ cup (59.15 ml) olive oil

Directions:

Whisk together all ingredients.

Nutrition Facts	
Serving Size	2 Tablespoons

Amount Per Serving	
Calories	**180**

	Kidney Friendly % DV*
Total Fat 20g	25%
Saturated Fat 3g	17%
Trans Fat 0g	
Cholesterol 0mg	0%
Total Carbohydrate 1g	0%
Dietary Fiber 0g	0%
Total Sugars 11g	
Includes 0g Added Sugar	0%
Protein 0g	
Sodium 185mg	8%
Potassium 20mg	1%
Phosphorus 0mg	0%
ORAC 440	1%
Polyphenols 15mg	2%
AGE	LOW
PRAL	-0.4
Dietary Nitrates	LOW

* The % Daily Value (DV) tells you how much a nutrient in a serving of food contributes to the daily kidney friendly diet. 2,000 calories a day is used for general nutrition advice.

Lemon-Herb Vinaigrette

Makes about ⅓ cup

Ingredients:

1 clove garlic, minced

1 teaspoon (5.19 g) Dijon mustard

1 teaspoon (2 g) lemon zest

¼ teaspoon (0.3 g) dried rosemary (or use ½ teaspoon fresh)

½ teaspoon (0.6 g) dried thyme (or use ½ teaspoon fresh)

1 tablespoon (15 g) fresh lemon juice

¼ teaspoon (1.42 g) salt

¼ teaspoon (0.57 g) pepper

¼ cup (59.15 ml) olive oil

Directions:

Whisk together all ingredients

Make Ahead: To make in advance, keep the salad, baked potato, and dressing separate until ready to serve.

Cost Analysis:

Sweet potatoes are running around $1.25 per lb, so assume half a pound for one sweet potato or $0.63 and another $1.00 for the salad for a total for $1.63.

Nutrition Facts	
Serving Size	2 Tablespoons

Amount Per Serving	
Calories	**180**

	Kidney Friendly % DV*
Total Fat 20g	25%
Saturated Fat 3g	14%
Trans Fat 0g	
Cholesterol 0mg	0%
Total Carbohydrate 1g	0%
Dietary Fiber 0g	0%
Total Sugars 11g	
Includes 0g Added Sugar	0%
Protein 0g	
Sodium 205mg	9%
Potassium 20mg	1%
Phosphorus 0mg	0%
ORAC 930	3%
Polyphenols 25mg	2%
AGE	LOW
PRAL	-0.4
Dietary Nitrates	LOW

* The % Daily Value (DV) tells you how much a nutrient in a serving of food contributes to the daily kidney friendly diet. 2,000 calories a day is used for general nutrition advice.

Pumpkin Soup with "Chorizo" Mushrooms & Corn

Prep Time: 20 minutes

Cook Time: 35 minutes

Serves 3

Zupas is a chain of healthy restaurants, and in the fall they have Pumpkin Chorizo soup. The soup is pretty amazing, but we need to eliminate the sausage, black beans, and salt. We can replace the chorizo with mushrooms and the black beans with corn. The Mrs. Dash line of Mexican and or fajita seasoning contains no salt and is available at most grocery stores or on Amazon.

Ingredients:

For the "chorizo":

1 tablespoon (13.63 g) olive oil

1½ cups (150 g) diced mushrooms (white or cremini)

½ cup (350 g) fresh or frozen (thawed) corn kernels

1 teaspoon (2.71 g) smoked paprika

¼ teaspoon (0.25 g) dried thyme

¼ teaspoon (0.25 g) garlic powder

⅛ teaspoon (0.12 g) ground cumin

⅛ teaspoon (0.28 g) black pepper

1 teaspoon or to taste salt-free Mexican or fajita seasoning (such as Mrs. Dash)

½ cup (13 g) crushed tortilla chips

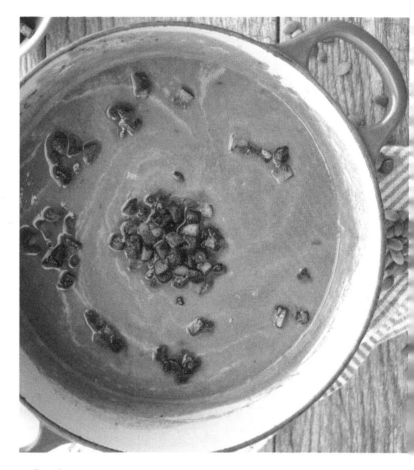

For the soup:

1 tablespoon (13.63 g) olive oil

2 cloves garlic, minced

2¼ cups (509 ml) salt-free vegetable broth

1½ cups (345 g) pumpkin puree

½ teaspoon (0.5 g) dried thyme

¼ teaspoon (0.25 g) garlic powder

¼ teaspoon (0.25 g) sweet or smoked paprika

1 cup (237 ml) unsweetened rice milk

3 tablespoons (44.37 ml) unsweetened coconut creamer (such as So Delicious)

Directions:

1. Heat 1 tablespoon oil in a saucepan over medium heat. Add the mushrooms and corn and sauté 8 to 10 minutes or until browned and tender. Remove from the pan and stir in the paprika, thyme, garlic powder, cumin, black pepper, and seasoning. Toss with the tortilla chips.

2. Add 1 tablespoon of olive oil the saucepan and return to medium heat. Add onion and sauté 5 to 7 minutes, or until the onion is soft. Add garlic and sauté 20 to 30 seconds or until fragrant. Stir in the vegetable broth, pumpkin, thyme, garlic powder, and paprika.

3. Bring to a boil, then reduce heat to medium-low. Simmer 7 to 10 minutes; stir in the rice milk and coconut creamer and cook 2 to 3 more minutes or until heated through. To serve, top with the corn and mushroom "chorizo."

Make Ahead: To make ahead, keep the chorizo and the soup separate until ready to serve.

Cost Analysis:

Like pumpkin chili, the actual cost for pumpkin will be less than $1.00 and up to $1.50 for the other ingredients, so $2.50.

Nutrition Facts	
Serving Size	1/3 Recipe

Amount Per Serving	
Calories	**275**

	Kidney Friendly % DV*
Total Fat 11g	15%
Saturated Fat 2g	9%
Trans Fat 0g	
Cholesterol 0mg	0%
Total Carbohydrate 43g	15%
Dietary Fiber 6g	19%
Total Sugars 11g	
Includes 0g Added Sugar	0%
Protein 6g	
Sodium 315mg	14%
Potassium 735mg	21%
Phosphorus 200mg	16%
ORAC 15180	51%
Polyphenols 620mg	62%
AGE	LOW
PRAL	-7.9
Dietary Nitrates	LOW

* The % Daily Value (DV) tells you how much a nutrient in a serving of food contributes to the daily kidney friendly diet. 2,000 calories a day is used for general nutrition advice.

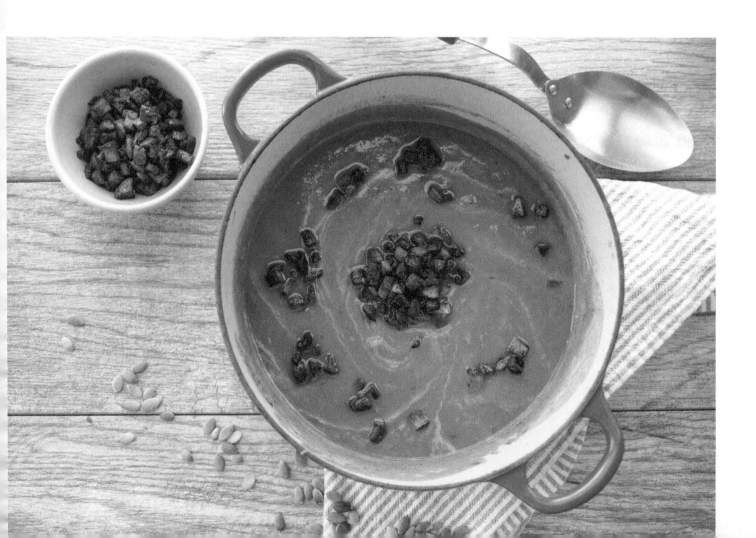

Thai Pineapple Salad with Carrot Cashew Dressing

Prep Time: 15 minutes

Cook Time: 5 minutes

Serves 2

This is a very refreshing treat from traditional salads. The mung bean noodles add calories and texture without adding protein.

Ingredients:

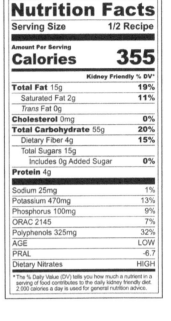

For the salad:

1 cup (70 g) thinly sliced cabbage

¾ cup (15 g) baby arugula

½ cup (90 g) thinly sliced red bell pepper

½ cucumber, cut into thin matchsticks

1 tablespoon (9.7 g) shredded carrot

½ cup (210 g) diced pineapple

1 tablespoon (8.6 g) coarsely chopped cashews

½ cup mung bean noodles, cooked

2 to 3 tablespoons (3 g) chopped fresh cilantro

Crushed red pepper, to taste

For the dressing:

1 tablespoon (8.6 g) chopped cashews

1 tablespoon (9.7 g) shredded carrot

1 clove garlic, minced

1 to 2 tablespoons (15 ml) water

1 tablespoon (13.63 g) sesame oil

1½ teaspoons (6.86 g) olive oil

1 tablespoon (15 g) fresh lime juice

Liquid stevia (to taste)

Directions:

1. For the dressing, combine all of the dressing ingredients in a blender and process until smooth.

2. Combine all of the salad ingredients except cilantro and crushed red pepper in a serving bowl; drizzle with dressing. Garnish with cilantro and crushed red pepper.

Cost Analysis:

We calculated $3.30 for this recipe when everything was added in.

Nutrition Facts	
Serving Size	1/2 Recipe
Amount Per Serving	
Calories	**355**
	Kidney Friendly % DV*
Total Fat 15g	19%
Saturated Fat 2g	11%
Trans Fat 0g	
Cholesterol 0mg	0%
Total Carbohydrate 55g	20%
Dietary Fiber 4g	15%
Total Sugars 15g	
Includes 0g Added Sugar	0%
Protein 4g	
Sodium 25mg	1%
Potassium 470mg	13%
Phosphorus 100mg	9%
ORAC 2145	7%
Polyphenols 325mg	32%
AGE	LOW
PRAL	-6.7
Dietary Nitrates	HIGH

* The % Daily Value (DV) tells you how much a nutrient in a serving of food contributes to the daily kidney friendly diet. 2,000 calories a day is used for general nutrition advice.

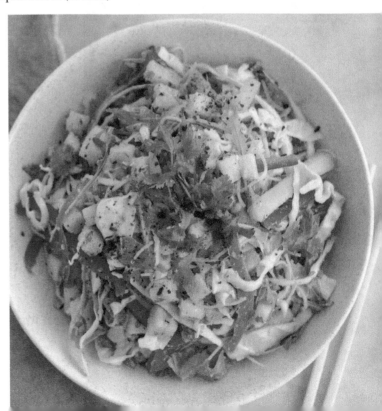

Vegetable Masala

Prep Time: 15 minutes

Cook Time: 5 minutes

Serves 2

This take on traditional Tikka Masala is packed with tons of fiber-rich vegetables, meaning you'll remain satisfied until dinner time.

Ingredients:

2 tablespoons (27.44 g) olive oil, divided

½ cup diced (75 g) onion

1 cup (200 g) chopped tomato

2 carrots, sliced (½ cup)(75 g)

1 teaspoon (2 g) minced fresh ginger

1 teaspoon (2.13 g) salt-free curry powder (such as McCormick)

¼ teaspoon (0.25 g) ground cumin

¼ teaspoon (0.25 g) ground coriander

3 cups (108 g) sliced collard greens

1 (13.5-ounce) can (398 ml) coconut milk

1 zucchini, sliced (1½ cups) (225 g)

1 (12-ounce) (340.19 g) package riced cauliflower* (see Note)

½ teaspoon (2.84 g) salt

½ teaspoon (1.14 g) pepper

¼ cup (4 g) fresh cilantro leaves

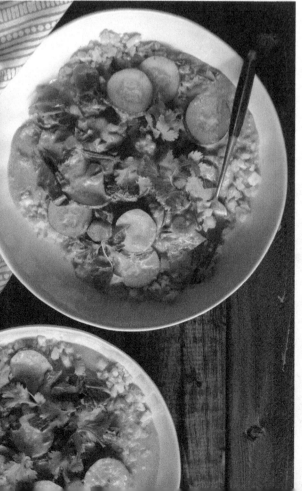

Directions:

1. Heat 1 tablespoon oil in a saucepan and sauté onion, tomato, carrot, ginger, and seasonings 5 minutes or until tender. (Puree with an immersion blender if you'd like a smoother curry.)

2. Add the collard greens and coconut milk and cook 5 minutes or until thickened. Add the zucchini and cook 3 minutes or just until tender. Season with ¼ teaspoon each salt and pepper.

3. Sauté the cauliflower in remaining 1 tablespoon oil until tender. Season with ¼ teaspoon salt and pepper. To serve, divide the cauliflower rice between serving bowls; top with the masala sauce and sprinkle with cilantro.

Note: Look for riced cauliflower in the produce department or freezer section of your grocery store. You may also grate 1 (12-ounce) package of cauliflower florets on a box grater to achieve riced cauliflower.

Make Ahead: Keep the masala, cauliflower rice, and cilantro separate until ready to serve.

Cost Analysis:

It seems most recipes are coming in around $3.00—this one is no exception.

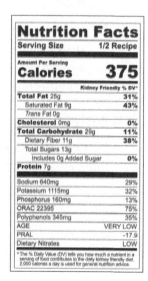

Nutrition Facts	
Serving Size	1/2 Recipe
Amount Per Serving	
Calories	**375**
	Kidney Friendly % DV*
Total Fat 25g	31%
Saturated Fat 9g	43%
Trans Fat 0g	
Cholesterol 0mg	0%
Total Carbohydrate 29g	11%
Dietary Fiber 11g	38%
Total Sugars 13g	
Includes 0g Added Sugar	0%
Protein 7g	
Sodium 640mg	29%
Potassium 1115mg	32%
Phosphorus 160mg	13%
ORAC 22395	75%
Polyphenols 346mg	35%
AGE	VERY LOW
PRAL	-17.9
Dietary Nitrates	LOW

* The % Daily Value (DV) tells you how much a nutrient in a serving of food contributes to the daily kidney friendly diet. 2,000 calories a day is used for general nutrition advice.

Gumbo Z'Herbes

Prep Time: 15 minutes

Cook Time: 30 minutes

Serves 2

Gumbo Z'Herbes or "Green Gumbo" is still served on Fridays at a handful of restaurants in New Orleans. Catholics giving up meat for Lent is what drove this tradition. The good news is this recipe is crazy healthy because the traditional roux is replaced by pureed vegetables for thickness. The bad news is it doesn't keep well even when frozen. My advice is to make on Fridays and enjoy on Saturday and Sunday. By Monday it will not taste so great.

Ingredients:

For the gumbo:

1 (12-ounce) (775 g) bunch collard greens, trimmed

2 tablespoons (27.44 g) olive oil

¼ cup onion, chopped (half reserved for garnish) (45 g)

1 green bell pepper, chopped (1 cup) (175 g)

1 stalk celery, chopped (¾ cup) (170 g)

1 clove garlic, minced

1 bay leaf

1 teaspoon (0.25 g) salt-free Cajun seasoning

½ teaspoon (2.84 g) salt

1 teaspoon (0.25 g) gumbo file powder (optional)

For the cauliflower rice:

1½ cups (250 g) riced cauliflower

1 teaspoon (4.57 g) olive oil

¼ teaspoon (1.42 g) salt

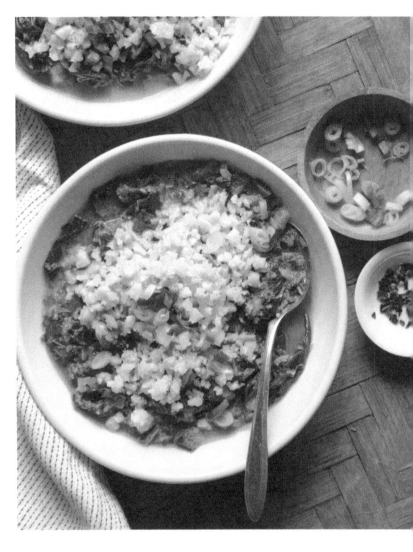

Nutrition Facts	
Serving Size	1/2 Recipe
Amount Per Serving	
Calories	**320**
	Kidney Friendly % DV*
Total Fat 19g	25%
Saturated Fat 3g	13%
Trans Fat 0g	
Cholesterol 0mg	0%
Total Carbohydrate 40g	14%
Dietary Fiber 18g	61%
Total Sugars 9g	
Includes 0g Added Sugar	0%
Protein 11g	
Sodium 465mg	21%
Potassium 1250mg	36%
Phosphorus 140mg	12%
ORAC 21420	71%
Polyphenols 620mg	62%
AGE	LOW
PRAL	-23..6
Dietary Nitrates	HIGH
* The % Daily Value (DV) tells you how much a nutrient in a serving of food contributes to the daily kidney friendly diet. 2,000 calories a day is used for general nutrition advice.	

Directions:

1. Rinse the collards well and chop. Place in a large pot and fill with water to cover. Simmer the collards 15 to 20 minutes or until tender. Drain the collards, reserving 1 cup cooking liquid. Let the collards cool slightly and chop into ½-inch pieces. Remove and puree half of the collards.

2. Heat the oil in a saucepan over medium heat; add the onion, 1 green onion, bell pepper, celery, and garlic. Cook 8 minutes or until very tender and beginning to caramelize. Remove half of the vegetables and puree.

3. Return the pureed vegetables to the pan. Add the 1 cup collard cooking liquid, bay leaf, Cajun seasoning, and salt. Stir in the pureed and chopped collards. Bring to a simmer and cook 10 minutes. Stir in the gumbo file powder (if using), and remove the bay leaf.

4. Saute the riced cauliflower in 1 teaspoon hot oil until tender. Stir in salt.

5. To serve, divide "gumbo" between 2 serving bowls. Top with a scoop of cauliflower rice, and garnish with remaining green onion.

Make Ahead: Keep the gumbo and cauliflower rice separate until ready to serve.

Cost Analysis:

Collard greens are less than $1.00 a bunch, but the peppers and rice cauliflower bring the total to around $2.75.

Portobello Steaks with Twice-Cooked Mashed Potatoes (or cauliflower) and Balsamic Arugula Salad

Prep Time: 20 minutes

Cook Time: 30 minutes

Serves 2

This was my go to recipe for comfort food or when I started dreaming about BBQ joints again. A trick for removing potassium from the potatoes is to slice them thinly for larger surface area and boiling and rinsing them twice. This can reduce the potassium by about 50%. This recipe is also a great make-ahead meal. Make the mushrooms in the beginning of the week and serve the extra portion when time is tight. It's not steak, but it's as close as we can get.

Ingredients:

For the portobello mushrooms:

4 large portobello mushrooms

1 cup (240 ml) red or white wine

2 tablespoons (28.3 g) balsamic vinegar

3 tablespoons (42.6 g) salt-free steak seasoning (such as Mrs. Dash)

2 tablespoons (27.44 g) olive oil

For the mashed potatoes:

4 pounds (1.81 kg) potatoes, peeled and thinly sliced

½ cup (113 g) unsalted butter (or use Smart Balance)

2 teaspoons (6.2 g) garlic powder

For the salad:

2 cups (40 g) arugula

1 small to medium tomato, cut into thick slices

1 teaspoon (5 g) balsamic vinegar

1 tablespoon (13.63 g) olive oil

Dash of oregano

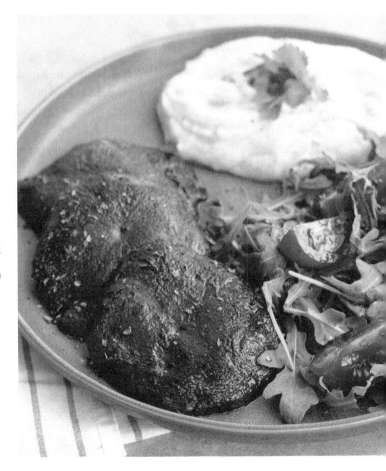

Directions:

1. Place the mushrooms in a sunny spot (like a windowsill) for one hour.

2. Remove the gills from the mushrooms with a spoon or dull knife; cut off stems. Wipe mushrooms with a paper towel and place in a large zip-top plastic bag. Stir together wine, vinegar, and seasoning. Pour over mushrooms in bag, and seal tightly. Set aside.

3. Meanwhile, make the mashed potatoes: Place the sliced potatoes in water to cover in a large saucepan; bring to a boil. Boil 15 minutes; drain potatoes and rinse with cold water.

4. Bring potatoes and more water to cover to a boil; cook 10 minutes, or until potatoes are tender. Drain potatoes, and rinse with water.

5. Return potatoes to the saucepan and add the butter and garlic powder. Mash with a potato masher or electric mixer to desired consistency.

6. Make the portobello mushrooms: Remove the mushrooms from the marinade and pat dry with a paper towel. Heat 2 tablespoons olive oil in a skillet and sauté mushrooms 5 to 6 minutes or until browned.

7. Make the salad: Combine the arugula and tomato. Whisk together the balsamic vinegar, oil, and oregano, and drizzle over the salad just before serving.

Cost Analysis:

Portobellos cost around $1.50 per large mushroom. Smaller ones will be cheaper and taste the same. The salad costs will be around $1.00, and the potatoes will cost $.50 to $.70 cents a pound. $3.00 per serving should cover it.

Nutrition Facts		
Serving Size One Serving of Each		
Amount Per Serving		
Calories		**625**
		Kidney Friendly % DV*
Total Fat 34g		44%
Saturated Fat 10g		51%
Trans Fat 0g		
Cholesterol 30mg		10%
Total Carbohydrate 65g		24%
Dietary Fiber 10g		34%
Total Sugars 10g		
Includes 0g Added Sugar		0%
Protein 12g		
Sodium 45mg		2%
Potassium 1765mg		50%
Phosphorus 365mg		30%
ORAC 6965		23%
Polyphenols 405mg		40%
AGE		LOW
PRAL		-21.8
Dietary Nitrates		MEDIUM

* The % Daily Value (DV) tells you how much a nutrient in a serving of food contributes to the daily kidney friendly diet. 2,000 calories a day is used for general nutrition advice.

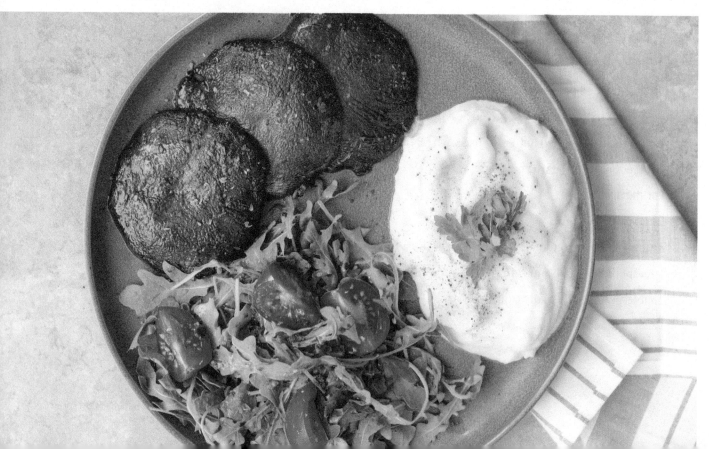

Pineapple and Vegetable Kebabs

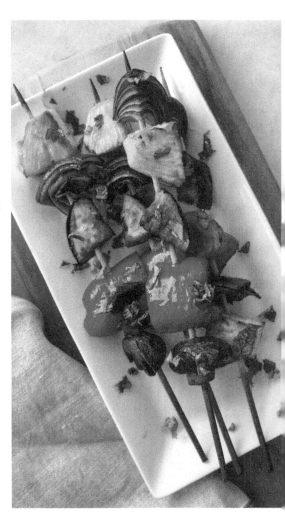

Prep Time: 20 minutes

Cook Time: 20 minutes

Serves 2

Grilling is part of summer and no one wants to feel left out. Combining this recipe with the charred Caesar salad and Strawberry Ice Cream (page 87) recipe are great for summer weekends. If you have guests eating meat, just add a few pieces of beef or chicken to the skewers. The flavor is great either way. The recipe here will be the indoor version, but you can grill as well.

Ingredients:

Wooden or metal skewers

1½ tablespoons (20.58 g) olive oil

1 tablespoon (16 g) No-Sodium Umami Sauce (see page 74)

¼ teaspoon (0.78 g) garlic powder

½ red onion, cut into wedges

½ cup (90 g) red bell pepper chunks

1 cup (82 g) eggplant chunks

1 cup (75 g) halved mushrooms

1 cup (165 g) pineapple chunks

1 to 2 tablespoons (6 g) chopped fresh cilantro

Directions:

1. If using wooden skewers, soak the wooden skewers in water for 20 minutes. Drain.

2. Preheat the oven to 400°F. Combine the olive oil, garlic powder, and a pinch of salt in a bowl. Add the onion, bell pepper, eggplant, mushrooms, and pineapples and toss to coat.

3. Thread the vegetables and pineapple onto the skewers and arrange on a parchment-lined baking sheet.

4. Bake the skewers for 10 minutes; turn and cook 10 more minutes.

5. Increase the oven temperature to broil. Broil the skewers 1 to 2 minutes or until the vegetables and pineapple are charred (watch them carefully to prevent burning). Remove from the oven and serve.

Cost Analysis:

This one is pretty cheap with every version coming in under $2.00 per serving.

Nutrition Facts		
Serving Size		1/2 Recipe
Amount Per Serving		
Calories		**205**
		Kidney Friendly % DV*
Total Fat 12g		16%
Saturated Fat 2g		11%
Trans Fat 0g		
Cholesterol 0mg		0%
Total Carbohydrate 25g		9%
Dietary Fiber 7g		23%
Total Sugars 13g		
Includes 0g Added Sugar		0%
Protein 4g		
Sodium 15mg		1%
Potassium 600mg		17%
Phosphorus 90mg		7%
ORAC 2280		8%
Polyphenols 290mg		29%
AGE		LOW
PRAL		-8.5
Dietary Nitrates		LOW

* The % Daily Value (DV) tells you how much a nutrient in a serving of food contributes to the daily kidney friendly diet. 2,000 calories a day is used for general nutrition advice.

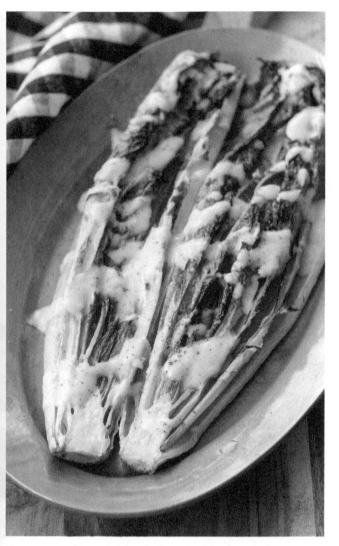

Charred Romaine with Caesar Dressing

Prep Time: 10 minutes

Cook Time: 5 minutes

Serves 1

The idea of grilling or cooking lettuce was foreign to me until we tried this recipe. Just about every guest will like this recipe if you are grilling. It's also cheap and low in potassium to offset the rest of the menu.

Ingredients:

1 head romaine lettuce

1½ tablespoons (20.58 g) olive oil, divided

1½ tablespoons (22.5 g) fresh lemon juice

¼ cup (33.5 g) chopped macadamia nuts, toasted

¼ teaspoon (1.25 g) Dijon mustard

¼ teaspoon (0.78 g) ground cumin

1½ teaspoons (7.5 ml) water

¼ teaspoon (0.70 g) minced garlic

Pinch of black pepper

Directions:

1. Preheat the broiler. Cut the romaine in half lengthwise. Rub ½ tablespoon of olive oil all over both halves. Broil the romaine on the top oven rack 1 to 2 minutes on each side. (You can also grill the romaine 1 to 2 minutes on each side if you'd like.)

2. Combine the remaining 1 tablespoon oil, lemon juice, macadamia nuts, mustard, cumin, 1 ½ teaspoons water, and garlic in a blender; process until smooth. Drizzle over the romaine halves and top with black pepper.

Cost Analysis:

A pack of six romaine hearts cost $3.98 at my local store. If we add dressing costs, we are still around $1.00 per serving.

Nutrition Facts

Serving Size	Entire Recipe

Amount Per Serving

Calories	540

	Kidney Friendly % DV*
Total Fat 48g	62%
Saturated Fat 7g	35%
Trans Fat 0g	
Cholesterol 0mg	0%
Total Carbohydrate 28g	10%
Dietary Fiber 17g	55%
Total Sugars 13g	
Includes 0g Added Sugar	0%
Protein 11g	

Sodium 70mg	3%
Potassium 1720mg	49%
Phosphorus 260mg	22%
ORAC 800	27%
Polyphenols 510mg	51%
AGE	LOW
PRAL	-29
Dietary Nitrates	VERY HIGH

* The % Daily Value (DV) tells you how much a nutrient in a serving of food contributes to the daily kidney friendly diet. 2,000 calories a day is used for general nutrition advice.

Jackfruit "Carnitas" Tacos

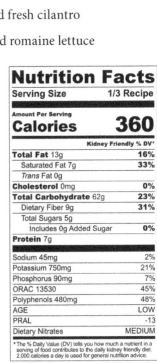

Prep Time: 15 minutes

Cook Time: 20 minutes

Serves 3

Jackfruit will be new to many of you. Jackfruit is very common in Asia but just starting to show up in the states. It takes on the flavor of the sauce in most cases and works great as a substitute for pork and crab cakes. If you can find fresh jackfruit, it works best (we like to order Edward and Sons from Amazon), but you can find canned as well, in Asian grocery stores or online. When buying canned jackfruit be sure to buy it packed in water, not brine.

Ingredients:

1 pound (302 g) fresh young jackfruit pieces (about 2 cups)

2 tablespoons (28.3 g) olive oil

1 cup (150 g) diced red onion

½ teaspoon (1.55 g) garlic powder

1 tablespoon (8.12 g) chili powder

1 teaspoon (3.1 g) ground cumin

1 teaspoon (3.1 g) paprika

½ teaspoon (0.5 g) dried oregano

½ teaspoon (2.6 g) apple cider vinegar

1½ cups (375 ml) salt-free vegetable broth

½ green bell pepper, thinly sliced

9 corn tortillas, warmed

2 tablespoons (6 g) chopped fresh cilantro

1½ cups (115 g) thinly sliced romaine lettuce

½ lime, cut into sections

Nutrition Facts		
Serving Size		1/3 Recipe
Amount Per Serving		
Calories		**360**
		Kidney Friendly % DV*
Total Fat 13g		**16%**
Saturated Fat 7g		33%
Trans Fat 0g		
Cholesterol 0mg		**0%**
Total Carbohydrate 62g		**23%**
Dietary Fiber 9g		31%
Total Sugars 5g		
Includes 0g Added Sugar		0%
Protein 7g		
Sodium 45mg		2%
Potassium 750mg		21%
Phosphorus 90mg		7%
ORAC 13530		45%
Polyphenols 480mg		48%
AGE		LOW
PRAL		-13
Dietary Nitrates		MEDIUM

* The % Daily Value (DV) tells you how much a nutrient in a serving of food contributes to the daily kidney friendly diet. 2,000 calories a day is used for general nutrition advice.

Directions:

1. Rinse and drain the jackfruit. (If you are using packaged jackfruit, rinse and place in a bowl or jar with enough water to cover and let stand in the refrigerator overnight. Drain, rinse, and drain the jackfruit.) (If you are using canned jackfruit, drain and rinse the jackfruit. Place the pieces in a bowl or jar with enough water to cover and let stand in the refrigerator for 6 hours. Drain and rinse the jackfruit, then repeat the soaking process 1-2 more times.)

2. Heat the oil in a saucepan over medium heat until hot; add the red onion. Sauté for 3 minutes, then add the spices, apple cider vinegar, and tomato paste, if using. Stir for 15-30 seconds, then stir in the drained jackfruit. Add the broth and bring to a boil; cover, reduce heat, and simmer for 15 minutes. Uncover, and stir in the sliced peppers. Cover and cook on medium-low heat for another 10-15 minutes. (If the liquid is evaporating too quickly, add an additional ¼ cup of broth.) Remove the pan from the heat and shred the jackfruit pieces using two forks; stir in cilantro. Serve on top of warmed tortillas with shredded lettuce.

Cost Analysis:

Shredded jackfruit runs the price up a little to $3.50 per serving.

Tortilla Soup

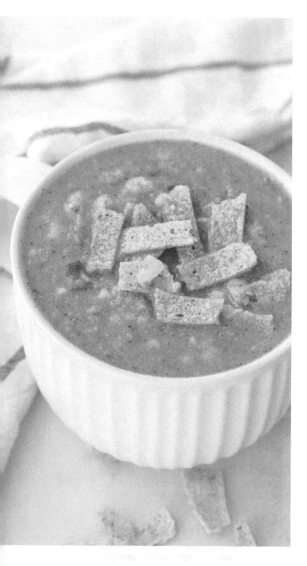

Prep Time: 15 minutes

Cook Time: 20 minutes

Serves 2

Tortilla soup is not exactly a health food, but it does satisfy cravings for those of us from border states. It's great on a cold day.

Ingredients:

1 tablespoon (13.72 g) olive oil

½ cup (75 g) chopped onion

½ cup (90 g) chopped green bell pepper

½ cup (90 g) chopped red bell pepper

3 cloves garlic, minced

½ teaspoon (1.35 g) chili powder

¼ to ½ teaspoon (0.77 g) ground cumin

¼ teaspoon (0.77 g) paprika

¼ teaspoon (0.25 g) dried oregano

1½ cups (265 g) frozen corn kernels, thawed

1 cup (132 g) frozen cauliflower florets, thawed

2 ½ cups (625 ml) salt-free vegetable broth

1 cup of unsalted tortilla chips

Nutrition Facts	
Serving Size	1/2 Recipe
Amount Per Serving	
Calories	**310**
	Kidney Friendly % DV*
Total Fat 12g	16%
Saturated Fat 4g	20%
Trans Fat 0g	
Cholesterol 0mg	0%
Total Carbohydrate 53g	19%
Dietary Fiber 10g	34%
Total Sugars 13g	
Includes 0g Added Sugar	0%
Protein 7g	
Sodium 30mg	1%
Potassium 625mg	18%
Phosphorus 165mg	14%
ORAC 24565	82%
Polyphenols 915mg	92%
AGE	LOW
PRAL	-7.1
Dietary Nitrates	LOW

* The % Daily Value (DV) tells you how much a nutrient in a serving of food contributes to the daily kidney friendly diet. 2,000 calories a day is used for general nutrition advice.

Directions:

1. Heat the oil in a saucepan over medium heat until hot. Add the onion, green bell pepper, and red bell peppers. Sauté 5 minutes or until the vegetables are softened. Add garlic and stir until fragrant, about 30 seconds. Stir in chili powder, cumin, paprika, and oregano.

2. Remove two-thirds of the vegetables from the pan and set aside. Add the corn, cauliflower, and vegetable broth to the remaining vegetables in the pan and bring to a boil. Cover, reduce heat, and simmer until the cauliflower is fork-tender.

3. Remove about half of the veggies using a ladle (it doesn't need to be perfect, just remove some and leave some left in the pot. Use an immersion blender or standard blender to puree the soup to desired consistency.

4. Return the reserved vegetables to the saucepan and cook over medium-low heat for 5 more minutes. If the soup is too thick, add additional vegetable broth until the desired consistency is reached. Remove the soup from the heat, and stir in the cilantro. Top the soup with tortilla chips and serve.

Cost Analysis:

Our cost was right at $1.50 per serving.

Ginger-Garlic Vegetable Ramen Bowls

Prep Time: 15 minutes

Cook Time: 20 minutes

Serves 2

Ramen bowls are easy, fast, and satisfying. For me, the umami sauce needs a little salt to taste right. While we are all on a low salt diet, if you have not added salt to any other meals, you can add a little salt to taste. Soy, teriyaki, and tamari all have loads of salt even the low salt versions. Just don't go overboard adding salt to taste.

Ingredients:

1 (4-ounce) (141 g) package mung bean noodles

1 tablespoon (13.72 g) sesame oil

1 tablespoon (13.72 g) vegetable oil

1 (8-ounce) (226.8 g) package sliced mushrooms

1 teaspoon (2 g) grated fresh ginger

2 cloves garlic, minced

1½ cups (105 g) tricolor coleslaw

1 cup (150 g) snow peas

¼ tsp (0.6 g) crushed red pepper

3 cups (715 ml) salt-free vegetable broth

2 tablespoons (30 ml) No-Sodium Umami Sauce (see below)

Garnish: sliced green onions and fresh basil

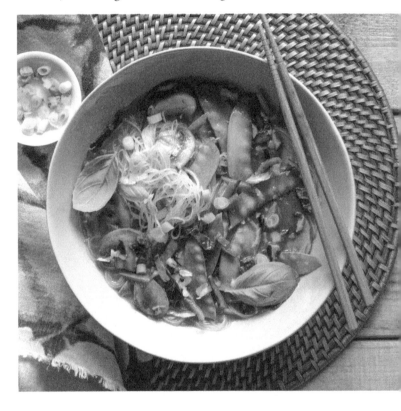

Directions:

1. Cook mung bean noodles according to package directions.

2. Heat the oil in a large saucepan over medium-high heat. Add mushrooms and sauté 6 minutes or until browned and tender. Stir in the ginger and garlic. Cook 2 minutes longer.

3. Add the coleslaw, snow peas, and crushed red pepper. Cook 3 minutes or until vegetables soften. Add the vegetable broth and Umami Sauce.

4. To serve, divide noodles evenly between 2 bowls. Top with broth mixture and garnish with green onion and basil.

Nutrition Facts		
Serving Size		1/2 Recipe
Amount Per Serving		
Calories		**520**
		Kidney Friendly % DV*
Total Fat 16g		21%
Saturated Fat 4g		20%
Trans Fat 0g		
Cholesterol 0mg		0%
Total Carbohydrate 88g		32%
Dietary Fiber 11g		37%
Total Sugars 8g		
Includes 0g Added Sugar		0%
Protein 8g		
Sodium 40mg		1%
Potassium 960mg		28%
Phosphorus 230mg		19%
ORAC 2570		9%
Polyphenols 100mg		10%
AGE		VERY LOW
PRAL		-10
Dietary Nitrates		MEDIUM

* The % Daily Value (DV) tells you how much a nutrient in a serving of food contributes to the daily kidney friendly diet. 2,000 calories a day is used for general nutrition advice.

No-Sodium Umami Sauce

This recipe is adapted from the blog Gluten Free & More.

Ingredients:

½ cup (115 ml) water

1 1 ½ teaspoons (7.5 g) rice vinegar

½ teaspoon (3.59 g) molasses

¼ teaspoon (1.04 g) brown sugar

¼ teaspoon (0.78 g) garlic powder

Directions:

Stir together all ingredients in a jar. Refrigerate for up to 1 month.

Cost Analysis:

Mung bean noodles cost less than $0.25 per serving, and pre-packaged shredded cabbage is around $1.67 for a 16-ounce package. No-salt broth can be found most anywhere today, and will cost around $3.00 per 16-ounce container. Again, we are less than $3.00 per serving.

Main Dish Salad

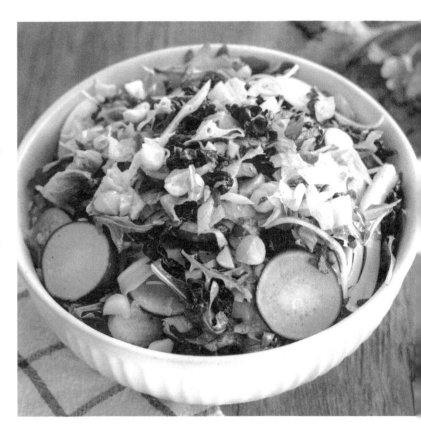

Prep Time: 15 minutes

Serves 2

In the raw food community, large salads with a wide variety of ingredients are a staple. You can add just about any ingredient you want within reason. There is no reason to limit what you put these salads that serve as a main course meal. Adding crunchy and chewy foods to the mix will make it more satisfying. Adding herbs like basil or mint are also great ideas.

Ingredients:

For the Dressing:

2 tablespoons (30 g) fresh lemon juice

3 tablespoons (40.89 g) olive oil

1 clove garlic, minced

1 teaspoon (5 g) Dijon mustard

¼ teaspoon (0.57 g) pepper

1 teaspoon (7.08 g) honey

For the Salad:

3 cups (230 g) thinly sliced romaine lettuce

2 cups (40 g) arugula

1 cup (20 g) watercress

2 tablespoons (16.75 g) chopped macadamia nuts or pecans

2 tablespoons (15 g) reduced-sugar dried cranberries

2 tablespoons (6 g) chopped fresh parsley or cilantro

½ cup (60 g) chopped fruit (such as apples, pears, or berries)

Fresh basil or mint (optional)

Nutrition Facts	
Serving Size	1/2 Recipe
Amount Per Serving	
Calories	**305**
	Kidney Friendly % DV*
Total Fat 27g	35%
Saturated Fat 4g	19%
Trans Fat 0g	
Cholesterol 0mg	0%
Total Carbohydrate 17g	6%
Dietary Fiber 6g	20%
Total Sugars 7g	
Includes 3g Added Sugar	6%
Protein 3g	
Sodium 50mg	2%
Potassium 525mg	15%
Phosphorus 75mg	6%
ORAC 3680	12%
Polyphenols 210mg	21%
AGE	LOW
PRAL	-9.4
Dietary Nitrates	HIGH

*The % Daily Value (DV) tells you how much a nutrient in a serving of food contributes to the daily kidney friendly diet. 2,000 calories a day is used for general nutrition advice.

Directions:

1. To make the dressing, combine all of the ingredients in a jar. Seal and shake well until the dressing is well combined.

2. Combine all of the salad ingredients in a large bowl. Toss with the dressing, and enjoy.

Cost Analysis:

Like other recipes in this chapter, the cost is still under $3.00 per serving.

Mushroom Bourguignon

Prep Time: 15 minutes

Cook Time: 30 minutes

Serves 2

This dish is excellent for the "foodie" in your house who is trying to limit protein. It's something a little French and hearty, and is another great meat substitute. When I was making the change, I focused on hearty meals that satisfy my cravings for meat. This one is a little involved to prepare, but worth it if you are a fan of these kinds of foods. Toasted French bread is a great side, see next page on bread.

Ingredients:

1 tablespoon (13.63 g) olive oil

1 tablespoon (14.2 g) real butter or butter substitute (such as Smart Balance)

½ cup (75 g) diced red onion

½ cup (25 g) diced carrots

⅔ cup (150 g) diced celery

3 cloves garlic, minced

1 teaspoon (0.91 g) dried thyme

1 (8-ounce) (226.8 g) package sliced mushrooms, diced

1 tablespoon (16.61 g) tomato paste

½ cup (120 ml) dry red wine

1 cup (240 ml) salt-free vegetable broth

2 ounces (56.7 g) sliced mushrooms

½ tablespoon (4 g) arrowroot or tapioca starch

¼ teaspoon (0.57 g) pepper

1 to 2 tablespoons (6 g) chopped fresh parsley

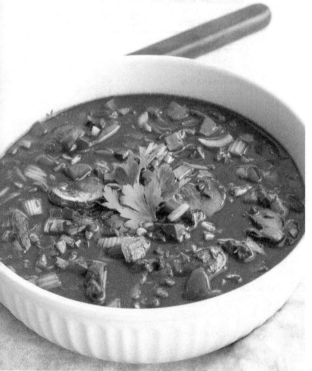

Directions:

1. Heat the olive oil and butter in a saucepan over medium heat, and cook until the butter melts. Add the onion, carrots, and celery, and sauté for 5 minutes. Add the garlic and thyme and stir until fragrant. Add the diced mushrooms and sauté for 1 minute, then add the tomato paste and red wine. Bring to a boil; stir in the broth. Return to a boil; cover, reduce the heat and simmer for 10 minutes. Uncover and add the sliced mushrooms and cook for 2-3 minutes, stirring occasionally.

2. In a small bowl, whisk together the arrowroot or tapioca starch and 2 tablespoons of broth from the saucepan to make a slurry. Stir the slurry into the mushroom mixture. Cook for 2-3 minutes until the liquid has slightly thickened and the sliced mushrooms are tender. Remove from the heat, and stir in the black pepper and parsley before serving.

Nutrition Facts

Serving Size	1/2 Recipe

Amount Per Serving	
Calories	**255**

	Kidney Friendly % DV*
Total Fat 13g	17%
Saturated Fat 5g	23%
Trans Fat 0g	
Cholesterol 15mg	5%
Total Carbohydrate 22g	8%
Dietary Fiber 6g	19%
Total Sugars 7g	
Includes 0g Added Sugar	0%
Protein 6g	

Sodium 95mg	4%
Potassium 1190mg	34%
Phosphorus 250mg	21%
ORAC 6180	21%
Polyphenols 265mg	26%
AGE	LOW
PRAL	-15
Dietary Nitrates	MEDIUM

* The % Daily Value (DV) tells you how much a nutrient in a serving of food contributes to the daily kidney friendly diet. 2,000 calories a day is used for general nutrition advice.

Cost Analysis:

While this recipe is a little more involved than most, but the cost comes in at $3.25 per serving.

Bread

While bread is a great side for many recipes like bourguignon, bread is not exactly a health food for us. Bread has high protein in relationship to the number of calories, a positive acid load and is low in nutrients compared to many foods. What is the answer for bread lovers who need to lower protein?

The answer is a woman named Malathy Ramanujam. Her son was diagnosed with a rare disease that limits his daily protein intake. Again, patients and family members can do remarkable things. There are many low protein bread or mixes on the market. However, we think Malathy's is the best. For the record, I don't know Malathy personally and have no business relationship with her.

I am listing Malathy's because I think her mixes and recipes will get your closest to the bread you are used to eating. We used a bread maker and you may want to invest in one. It's the easiest way by far. Prices have come down and now you can find bread makers in the $50 to $70 range.

Malathy's website is www.tasteconnections.com. You will find mixes for: bread, baking mixes, tapioca popcorn and a few others. I am no expert in baking or bread making, so I would refer all questions to her site: www.tasteconnections.com

Low protein baking mix

Nutrition Facts

Serving Size	1 Cup (110g)

Amount Per Serving

Calories 420

	% Daily Value*
Total Fat 8g	10%
Saturated Fat 1g	5%
Trans Fat 0g	
Cholesterol 0mg	0%
Sodium 460mg	19%
Total Carbohydrate 89g	32%
Dietary Fiber 4g	13%
Total Sugars 2g	
Includes 0g Added Sugar	0%
Protein 0g	
Vitamin D 2mcg	0%
Calcium 260mg	0%
Iron 0.7mg	4%
Potassium 0mg	0%

*The % Daily Value (DV) tells you how much a nutrient in a serving of food contributes to a daily diet. 2,000 calories a day is used for general nutrition advice.

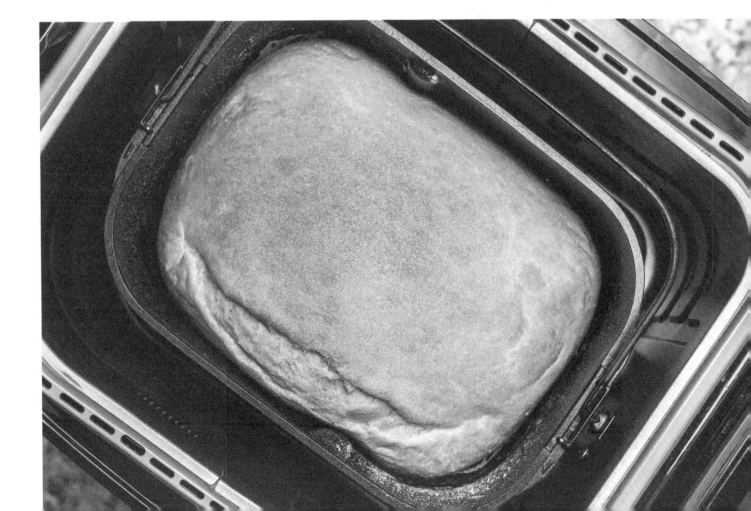

Pepper Salad

Prep Time: 15 minutes

Cook Time: 30 minutes

Serves 2

Tapas bars popped up in every major city in the 1990's. Tapas are small savory dishes served at bars in Spain. For me, tapas translated to incredibly expensive appetizers. You can have tapas night at home, eat well and save your money. The pepper salad, marinated carrots and watermelon gazpacho go together to make a meal. Make these ahead of time so they can marinade a little longer. If you are grilling over the weekend, these also make great appetizers.

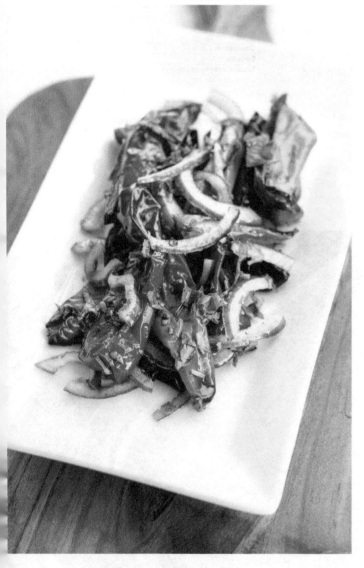

Ingredients:

1 (8-ounce) (225 g) package mixed mini sweet peppers

1½ tablespoons (20.45 g) olive oil, divided

½ cup thinly (75 g) sliced red onions

1 tablespoon (6 g) minced fresh parsley or cilantro

1 teaspoon (4.76 g) red wine vinegar

Directions:

1. Preheat the oven to 400°F. Halve and seed the peppers. Toss with 1 tablespoon of olive oil until well coated. Line a sheet pan with parchment paper, and arrange the peppers, cut-sides-down on the pan. Bake for 15 minutes, then flip the peppers over. Return to the oven and bake until the peppers are browned or charred to desired doneness. Remove from the oven and let cool.

2. In a bowl, combine the red onion, parsley or cilantro, red wine vinegar, and remaining ½ tablespoon olive oil. Add the peppers and toss gently.

Cost Analysis:

A bag of small red, yellow, and orange peppers is $2.98 at my local store.

Nutrition Facts	
Serving Size	1/2 Recipe
Amount Per Serving	
Calories	**130**
	Kidney Friendly % DV*
Total Fat 11g	**14%**
Saturated Fat 1.5g	**8%**
Trans Fat 0g	
Cholesterol 0mg	**0%**
Total Carbohydrate 11g	**4%**
Dietary Fiber 4g	**12%**
Total Sugars 6g	
Includes 0g Added Sugar	**0%**
Protein 2g	
Sodium 10mg	0%
Potassium 365mg	10%
Phosphorus 45mg	4%
ORAC 1830	6%
Polyphenols 250mg	25%
AGE	LOW
PRAL	-6
Dietary Nitrates	LOW

* The % Daily Value (DV) tells you how much a nutrient in a serving of food contributes to the daily kidney friendly diet. 2,000 calories a day is used for general nutrition advice.

Watermelon Gazpacho

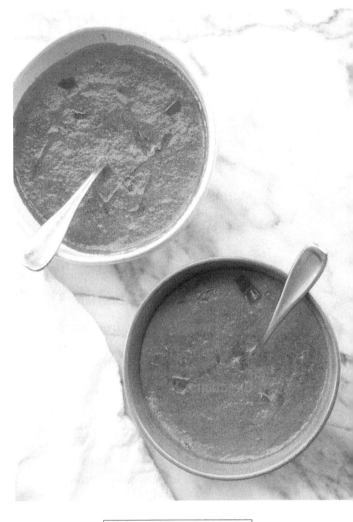

Prep Time: 10 minutes

Serves 2

Gazpacho is a cold tomato-based soup with a little kick to it. While cold soup may be an acquired taste for some, it's a very refreshing choice especially during hot summer months. Using watermelon and peppers in place of traditional tomatoes reduces the potassium. Watermelon is high in citrulline which increases nitric oxide.

Ingredients:

3 cups (456 g) chopped watermelon, divided

1 cup (180 g) chopped red bell pepper, divided

½ cup (52 g) chopped cucumber

2 tablespoons (12 g) chopped green onion(optional)

1 clove garlic, minced

1 tablespoon (14.3 g) red wine vinegar

2 tablespoons (27.26 g) olive oil

⅛ teaspoon (0.28 g) black pepper

Chopped green onion or fresh basil (for garnish), optional

Directions:

1. Combine 2½ cups of watermelon, ¾ cup red bell pepper, and the remaining ingredients in a high speed blender; process until smooth. Stir in the remaining watermelon and red bell pepper.

2. Divide soup among serving bowls. Drizzle with olive oil, and garnish with green onion or basil, if desired.

Cost Analysis:

Out-of-season seedless watermelons cost $7.99 in my area. Peppers and cucumber are $1.50 combined. You don't use all of the watermelon in this recipe, so the real cost is around $3.50 per serving.

Nutrition Facts	
Serving Size	1/2 Recipe
Amount Per Serving	
Calories	**225**
	Kidney Friendly % DV*
Total Fat 14g	**18%**
Saturated Fat 2g	**9%**
Trans Fat 0g	
Cholesterol 0mg	**0%**
Total Carbohydrate 25g	**9%**
Dietary Fiber 3g	**11%**
Total Sugars 18g	
Includes 0g Added Sugar	**0%**
Protein 3g	
Sodium 10mg	0%
Potassium 510mg	15%
Phosphorus 60mg	5%
ORAC 1485	5%
Polyphenols 340mg	34%
AGE	LOW
PRAL	-8.7
Dietary Nitrates	LOW

* The % Daily Value (DV) tells you how much a nutrient in a serving of food contributes to the daily kidney friendly diet. 2,000 calories a day is used for general nutrition advice.

Marinated Carrot Salad

Prep Time: 10 minutes

Cook Time: 5 minutes

Serves 3

Of all the tapas recipes we tried, this was the clear winner on our household. It's simple, easy, and good for you.

Ingredients:

3 cups (150 g) peeled and sliced carrots

1 to 2 cloves garlic, grated

2 tablespoons (0.1 g) chopped fresh dill

2 tablespoons (27.26 g) olive oil

2 teaspoons (30 g) fresh lemon juice

Pinch of black pepper

Directions:

1. Steam the carrots until just tender. Let cool for 15-20 minutes.

2. Combine the garlic, dill, olive oil, lemon juice, and black pepper in a bowl. Add the carrots and toss to coat. Let marinate in the refrigerator for a few hours before enjoying.

Cost Analysis:

A bag of prewashed and peeled baby carrots is less than $2.00

Nutrition Facts	
Serving Size	1/3 Recipe
Amount Per Serving	
Calories	**100**
	Kidney Friendly % DV*
Total Fat 8g	11%
Saturated Fat 1g	6%
Trans Fat 0g	
Cholesterol 0mg	0%
Total Carbohydrate 6g	2%
Dietary Fiber 1g	5%
Total Sugars 3g	
Includes 0g Added Sugar	0%
Protein 1g	
Sodium 35mg	2%
Potassium 180mg	5%
Phosphorus 20mg	2%
ORAC 635	2%
Polyphenols 45mg	4%
AGE	LOW
PRAL	-3.2
Dietary Nitrates	HIGH

* The % Daily Value (DV) tells you how much a nutrient in a serving of food contributes to the daily kidney friendly diet. 2,000 calories a day is used for general nutrition advice.

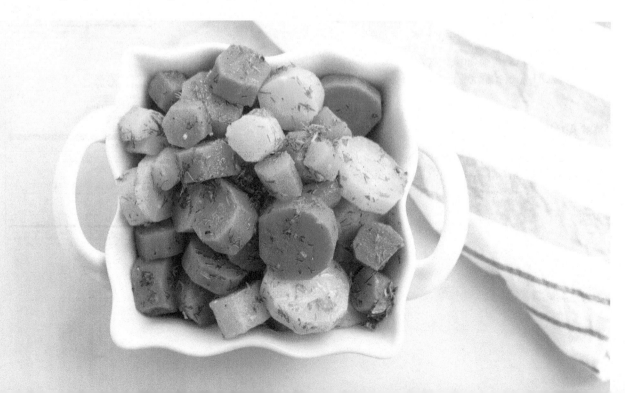

Jackfruit Crab Cakes

Prep Time: 20 minutes

Cook Time: 20 minutes

Serves 3

This is for the seafood lover in all of us. These cakes could fool even the biggest of seafood lovers. For best results, shape the patties and then refrigerate 8 hours or overnight. It allows them to hold their shape as they are pan-fried. Trader Joes has these as well, but the sodium is a bit high. Pair with the remoulade and coleslaw recipes that follow to round out the meal.

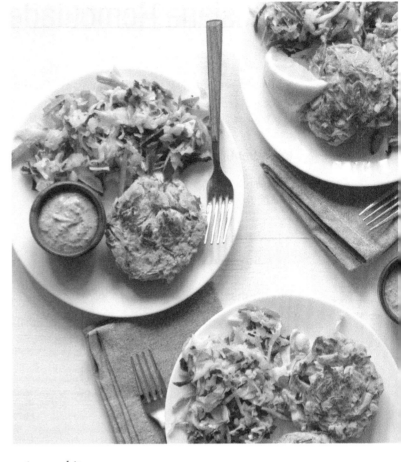

Ingredients:

2 (14-oz) (225 g) cans young jackfruit in water

1 teaspoon (4.57 g) olive oil

¼ cup (45 g) finely chopped red bell pepper

¼ cup (55 g) finely chopped celery

1 teaspoon (5 g) Dijon mustard

1 teaspoon (2 g) lemon zest

1 tablespoon (15 g) fresh lemon juice

3 tablespoons (21 g) coconut flour

½ teaspoon (0.75 g) paprika

½ teaspoon (1.55 g) garlic powder

Pinch of cayenne pepper

1 egg white

1 cup (100 g) steamed and mashed cauliflower (about 5 large florets)

1 green onion, chopped

1 tablespoon (13.72 g) olive oil

Directions:

1. Drain and rinse jackfruit; pat dry with paper towels and chop until it resembles crabmeat.

2. Sauté red bell pepper and celery in oil until tender.

3. Stir together mustard, lemon zest, lemon juice, coconut flour, paprika, garlic powder, cayenne pepper, and egg white in a bowl. Add jackfruit, cauliflower, bell pepper, and green onion.

4. Shape mixture into 6 patties and refrigerate overnight.

5. Coat "crab cakes" with nonstick spray. Heat 1 tablespoon oil in a large nonstick skillet. Cook 2 to 3 minutes on each side or until browned and warmed through. Serve with Remoulade.

Nutrition Facts	
Serving Size	1/3 Recipe
Amount Per Serving	
Calories	**235**
	Kidney Friendly % DV*
Total Fat 13g	**17%**
Saturated Fat 3g	**13%**
Trans Fat 0g	
Cholesterol 0mg	**0%**
Total Carbohydrate 28g	**10%**
Dietary Fiber 7g	**23%**
Total Sugars 2g	
Includes 0g Added Sugar	**0%**
Protein 6g	
Sodium 90mg	4%
Potassium 570mg	16%
Phosphorus 65mg	5%
ORAC 15635	52%
Polyphenols 130mg	13%
AGE	LOW
PRAL	-8.4
Dietary Nitrates	LOW

*The % Daily Value (DV) tells you how much a nutrient in a serving of food contributes to the daily kidney friendly diet. 2,000 calories a day is used for general nutrition advice.

Cost Analysis:

Jackfruit will cost between $3.00 and $4.00 a can. Assume $10.00 for everything or $3.33 per serving.

Louisiana Remoulade

Louisiana remoulade is what many of us are familiar with.   Classic french remoulade contains things like dill and capers. Louisiana remoulade is easy to make and tastes much better in my opinion. Remoulade also add needed calories, so indulge.

Ingredients:

¼ cup (56 g) Smart Balance mayonnaise

1 tablespoon (15 g) grainy mustard

1 teaspoon (1.5 g) paprika

1 teaspoon (5 g) prepared horseradish

Directions:

Stir together all ingredients. Refrigerate until ready to serve.

Cost Analysis:

Less than $1.00 per serving.

Nutrition Facts		
Serving Size		Entire Recipe
Amount Per Serving		
Calories		**210**
		Kidney Friendly % DV*
Total Fat 20g		26%
Saturated Fat 0g		0%
Trans Fat 0g		
Cholesterol 20mg		7%
Total Carbohydrate 10g		4%
Dietary Fiber 0g		3%
Total Sugars 2g		
Includes 0g Added Sugar		0%
Protein 1g		
Sodium 680mg		31%
Potassium 60mg		2%
Phosphorus 25mg		2%
ORAC 2140		7%
Polyphenols 45mg		5%
AGE		LOW
PRAL		-0.5
Dietary Nitrates		VERY LOW

* The % Daily Value (DV) tells you how much a nutrient in a serving of food contributes to the daily kidney friendly diet. 2,000 calories a day is used for general nutrition advice.

Vinegar Slaw

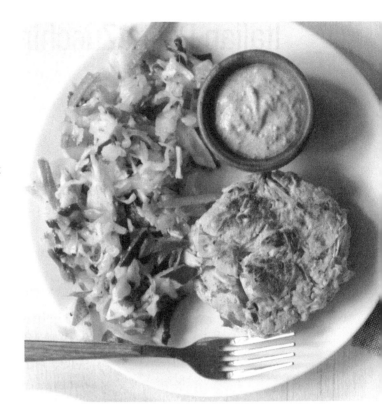

Prep Time: 10 minutes

Serves 3

This slaw can be made the day before or the day of. Just make sure you allow it to stand for at least 30 minutes to let the cabbage soften.

Ingredients:

4 cups (400 g) shredded tricolor coleslaw

¼ cup (5 g) chopped fresh parsley

2 tablespoons (28.6 g) apple cider vinegar

1 tablespoon (12.9 g) measures-like-sugar substitute

1 teaspoon (5 g) Dijon mustard

3 tablespoons (41.17 g) olive oil

¼ teaspoon (1.42 g) salt

¼ teaspoon (0.57 g) pepper

Directions:

Combine coleslaw, radishes, and parsley in a large bowl. Stir together vinegar, sugar substitute, mustard, olive oil, salt, and pepper. Pour over coleslaw mixture and toss to coat. Refrigerate at least 30 minutes to allow coleslaw to soften.

Cost Analysis:

A bag of tricolor coleslaw is $1.67 at my local store.

Nutrition Facts		
Serving Size		1/3 Recipe
Amount Per Serving		
Calories		**160**
		Kidney Friendly % DV*
Total Fat 14g		**18%**
Saturated Fat 2g		**10%**
Trans Fat 0g		
Cholesterol 0mg		**0%**
Total Carbohydrate 10g		**3%**
Dietary Fiber 2g		**7%**
Total Sugars 5g		
Includes 0g Added Sugar		**0%**
Protein 2g		
Sodium 240mg		11%
Potassium 265mg		8%
Phosphorus 40mg		3%
ORAC 1400		5%
Polyphenols 45mg		5%
AGE		LOW
PRAL		-4.4
Dietary Nitrates		HIGH

*The % Daily Value (DV) tells you how much a nutrient in a serving of food contributes to the daily kidney friendly diet. 2,000 calories a day is used for general nutrition advice.

Italian Pesto Zucchini Noodles

Prep Time: 20 minutes

Cook Time: 20 minutes

Serves 2

This Italian-inspired pasta dish features both mung bean noodles and zucchini noodles tossed with a creamy pesto sauce that you may want to keep in the fridge to use throughout the week when time is tight. Zucchini noodles always leave me hungry in an hour. Combining mung bean noodles solves the problem. Adding creamer add calories.

Ingredients:

1 (4-ounce) (141 g) package mung bean noodles

½ red bell pepper

2 cups zucchini noodles (9 ounces) (265 g)

3 tablespoons (41.17 g) olive oil, divided

½ teaspoon salt (2.84 g), divided

½ teaspoon (1.14 g) pepper, divided

1 tablespoon (15 g) fresh lemon juice

1 clove garlic, grated

½ cup (20.1 g) fresh basil

¼ cup (5 g) baby arugula

1½ teaspoons (7.5 ml) water

½ cup (120 ml) unsweetened coconut creamer (such as So Delicious)

1 teaspoon (2.5 g) cornstarch

Additional fresh or dried basil and crushed red pepper, for garnish

Directions:

1. Cook noodles according to package directions.

2. Broil red pepper until blackened (or place over a flame on a gas stovetop and turn with tongs); remove to a bowl and cover to allow steam to be trapped. Let stand 10 minutes; remove skin, seed and slice into strips. Sauté zucchini noodles in 1 tablespoon olive oil; season with ¼ teaspoon each salt and pepper.

3. Combine lemon juice, remaining 2 tablespoons olive oil, garlic, basil, kale, and water in a blender. Process until well blended. If the pesto is too thick, add a small amount of additional water to reach desired consistency.

4. Stir together coconut creamer and cornstarch. Cook over medium heat until thickened. Stir in pesto, and remaining ¼ teaspoon each salt and pepper. Toss with zucchini noodles and bell pepper.

5. Toss the noodles with the pesto cream. Top with fresh or dried basil and crushed red pepper, if desired.

Cost Analysis:

Again, this is another $3.00 meal.

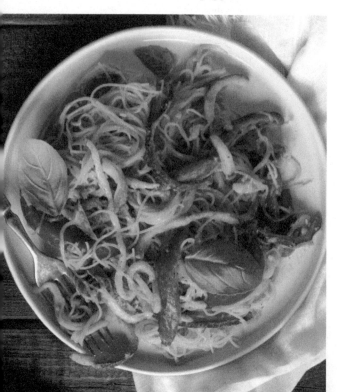

Nutrition Facts		
Serving Size		1/2 Recipe
Amount Per Serving		
Calories		**510**
		Kidney Friendly % DV*
Total Fat 23g		30%
Saturated Fat 5g		24%
Trans Fat 0g		
Cholesterol 0mg		0%
Total Carbohydrate 71g		26%
Dietary Fiber 3g		10%
Total Sugars 4g		
Includes 0g Added Sugar		0%
Protein 3g		
Sodium 575mg		26%
Potassium 475mg		14%
Phosphorus 90mg		8%
ORAC 2555		9%
Polyphenols 190mg		19%
AGE		VERY LOW
PRAL		-7.3
Dietary Nitrates		MEDIUM

* The % Daily Value (DV) tells you how much a nutrient in a serving of food contributes to the daily kidney friendly diet. 2,000 calories a day is used for general nutrition advice.

Vegetable Fajitas

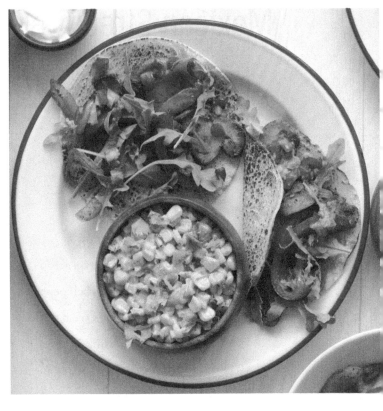

Prep Time: 10 minutes

Cook Time: 20 minutes

Serves 2

This dish is perfect for enjoying anytime of year. Combine with Mexican street corn for a meal. In the summer, toss the vegetables with the oil and cook in a grill basket. If the weather isn't optimal, sauté them in a skillet. For the meat eaters, add pork, chicken, steak, or shrimp to the mixture.

Ingredients:

For the fajitas:

1 tablespoon (13.72 g) olive oil

1 (8-ounce) (226.8 g) package sliced mushrooms

¼ teaspoon (1.42 g) salt

½ cup (90 g) sliced red bell pepper

½ cup (90 g) sliced green bell pepper

¼ cup (37.5 g) sliced onion

1 clove garlic, minced

½ teaspoon (1.56 g) ground cumin

½ teaspoon (1.56 g) chili powder

¼ teaspoon (0.25 g) dried oregano

6 corn tortillas, grilled or warmed

2 cups (40 g) baby arugula

2 tablespoons (30.25 g) sour cream

For the pico de gallo:

¼ cup (50 g) chopped tomato

2 tablespoons (6 g) chopped fresh cilantro

1 tablespoon (15 g) fresh lime juice

1 tablespoon (0.15 g) minced onion

Pinch of salt and pepper

Directions:

1. For the fajitas, heat the oil in a nonstick skillet over medium heat. Add the mushrooms and sprinkle with salt. Cover and cook 5 minutes or until the mushrooms are soft. Add the peppers and onion. Cover and cook 2 minutes or until the peppers and mushrooms soften. Uncover and cook 2 minutes or until vegetables begin to brown. Stir in garlic, cumin, chili powder, and oregano, and cook 2 minutes or until done.

2. Meanwhile, make the pico de gallo. Stir together all ingredients and set aside until ready to serve.

3. To serve, divide fajita vegetables evenly between tortillas and top with arugula, sour cream, and pico de gallo.

Cost Analysis:

Everyting combine came to $2.00 per serving, adding Mexican corn salad added 75 cents for a total of $2.75.

Nutrition Facts	
Serving Size	1/2 Recipe
Amount Per Serving	
Calories	**295**
	Kidney Friendly % DV*
Total Fat 13g	16%
Saturated Fat 4g	19%
Trans Fat 0g	
Cholesterol 0mg	0%
Total Carbohydrate 44g	16%
Dietary Fiber 9g	29%
Total Sugars 10g	
Includes 0g Added Sugar	0%
Protein 10g	
Sodium 355mg	16%
Potassium 1120mg	9%
Phosphorus 225mg	19%
ORAC 4135	14%
Polyphenols 565mg	57%
AGE	LOW
PRAL	-14.6
Dietary Nitrates	LOW

* The % Daily Value (DV) tells you how much a nutrient in a serving of food contributes to the daily kidney friendly diet. 2,000 calories a day is used for general nutrition advice.

Mexican Street Corn Salad

Prep Time: 10 minutes

Cook Time: 5 minutes

Serves 2

This side dish is great served warm or cold, meaning it's great to make early in the week and enjoy for lunches or to help save on dinnertime prep.

Ingredients:

1 tablespoon (13.72 g) olive oil

1½ cups (265 g) frozen corn kernels

¼ cup (45 g) chopped green bell pepper

2 tablespoons (6 g) chopped fresh cilantro

1 tablespoon (15 g) fresh lime juice

2 tablespoons (28 g) Smart Balance mayonnaise

½ teaspoon (0.5 g) paprika

¼ teaspoon (1.42 g) salt

¼ teaspoon (0.57 g) pepper

Directions:

1. Heat oil in a large skillet over medium-high heat. Add corn and bell pepper. Sauté 7 minutes or until tender and warmed through.

2. Stir together remaining ingredients. Add corn mixture, and toss to coat. Serve immediately or refrigerate until ready to serve.

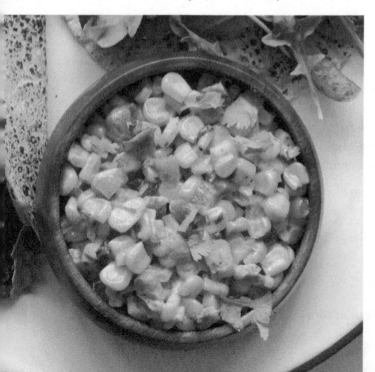

Cost Analysis:

$0.75 per serving.

Nutrition Facts

Serving Size	1/2 Recipe

Amount Per Serving	
Calories	**275**

	Kidney Friendly % DV*
Total Fat 13g	**17%**
Saturated Fat 1g	**7%**
Trans Fat 0g	
Cholesterol 5mg	**2%**
Total Carbohydrate 45g	**16%**
Dietary Fiber 9g	**31%**
Total Sugars 5g	
Includes 0g Added Sugar	**0%**
Protein 6g	
Sodium 415mg	19%
Potassium 510mg	15%
Phosphorus 120mg	10%
ORAC 22970	77%
Polyphenols 765mg	76%
AGE	LOW
PRAL	-6.5
Dietary Nitrates	LOW

* The % Daily Value (DV) tells you how much a nutrient in a serving of food contributes to the daily kidney friendly diet. 2,000 calories a day is used for general nutrition advice.

Strawberry (or Any Fruit) Ice Cream

Prep Time: 20 minutes

Cook Time: 40 minutes

Serves 6

My kids are hard to fool when it comes to ice cream, but as taste testers this one fooled them. Most dairy-free ice creams and sherbets are corn syrup-based which is a non starter for us. Other vegan ice creams are coconut milk-based and loaded with saturated fats. This recipe threads the needle by using rice milk, olive oil, and a lower amount of coconut milk. Canned coconut milk seems to work better than coconut cream. Use and spoon out the fat from canned coconut milk. (The can needs to be at room temperature or below before opening.) The watery portion can be used for something else later. Guar gum or pectin is available in most grocery stores. Ideally, you will add the highest antioxidant fruits in season you can find, but frozen varieties work just as well. Needless to say this recipe keeps well and can be frozen for long periods of time. If you like ice cream, buy an ice cream maker. It's worth it. You don't have to roast the berries, but it does help the flavor.

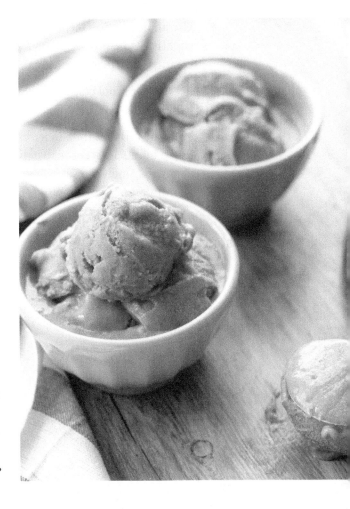

Ingredients:

1 pound (453.59 g) strawberries, halved (or use other fruit or berry)

1½ cups (375 ml) unenriched rice milk (such as Rice Dream)

6 tablespoons (90 ml) coconut milk

6 tablespoons (78 g) calorie-free sweetener

¼ teaspoon (0.07 g) guar gum or pectin

½ teaspoon (2.6 g) pure vanilla extract

2 tablespoons (27.44 g) olive oil

Directions:

1. Preheat the oven to 300°F. Place the strawberries, cut sides down on a rimmed baking sheet. Bake for 40 minutes.

2. Meanwhile, heat the rice milk and coconut milk in a small saucepan over medium heat. Stir in the sweetener and guar gum, and whisk until the milk mixture comes to a simmer.

3. Stir in the vanilla extract and roasted strawberries (along with any juices that have accumulated while roasting).

4. Use an immersion blender to puree in the saucepan or let cool slightly before processing in a stand blender. (For a sweeter ice cream, whisk in an additional 1 to 2 tablespoons sweetener.)

5. Let mixture cool completely. Stir in the olive oil and transfer to a freezer-safe container. Freeze 45 to 60 minutes.

6. Pour the mixture into an ice cream machine and process according to manufacturer's instructions. (The ice cream should take about 15 minutes to set). If necessary, freeze the ice cream 15 to 30 minutes before scooping.

Cost Analysis:

The cost will largely depend on the type of fruit or berry used in the recipe. Coconut milk will be about $1.00, rice milk another $1.00, and let's say the fruit is $4.00. $6.00 for six servings comes in at $1.00 per serving.

Nutrition Facts	
Serving Size	1/6 Recipe
Amount Per Serving	
Calories	**135**
	Kidney Friendly % DV*
Total Fat 9g	12%
Saturated Fat 4g	19%
Trans Fat 0g	
Cholesterol 0mg	0%
Total Carbohydrate 14g	5%
Dietary Fiber 2g	6%
Total Sugars 8g	
Includes 1g Added Sugar	2%
Protein 1g	
Sodium 30mg	1%
Potassium 175mg	5%
Phosphorus 50mg	4%
ORAC 3305	11%
Polyphenols 220mg	22%
AGE	LOW
PRAL	-2.2
Dietary Nitrates	HIGH

* The % Daily Value (DV) tells you how much a nutrient in a serving of food contributes to the daily kidney friendly diet. 2,000 calories a day is used for general nutrition advice.

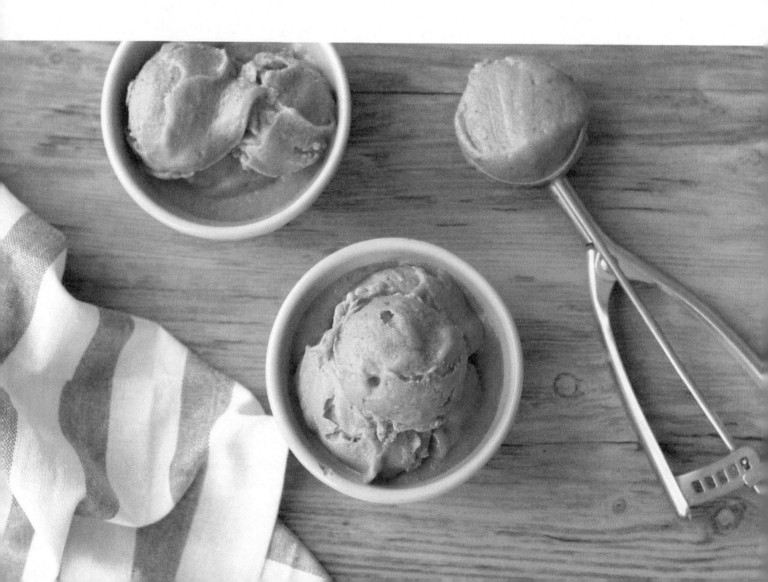

Watermelon-Blueberry Sorbet

Prep Time: 20 minutes

Serves 2

I was suspect of combining watermelon and blueberries. I felt like I was breaking some unknown food law. However, it is hard to argue with the results. Watermelon is high in citrulline which increases nitric oxide, and blueberries are high in antioxidants. The strawberry ice cream recipe has a vice of saturated fat, but this recipe does not. This one is actually guilt-free.

Ingredients:

2½ cups (380 g) seedless watermelon chunks

¼ cup (60 ml) water

½ cup (75 g) blueberries

3 tablespoons (38.7 g) calorie-free sweetener

1 teaspoon of pectin

Directions:

1. Process all of the ingredients in a blender or with an immersion blender until smooth.

2. Pour the mixture into a freezer-safe container and place in the freezer. Stir the mixture every hour until it reaches the desired consistency. Scoop into bowls and serve.

Cost Analysis:

The watermelon and blueberry cost come to just under $2.50. Each serving will cost $1.25.

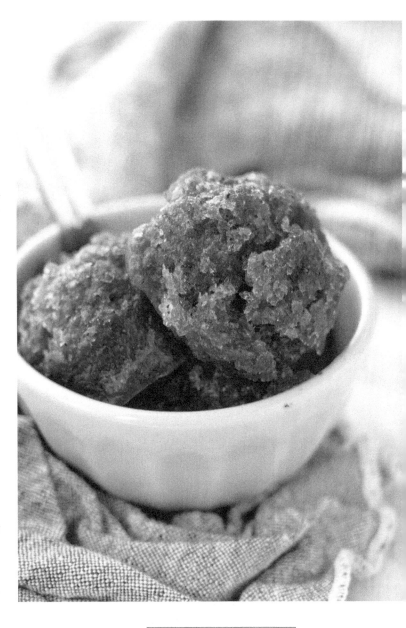

Nutrition Facts	
Serving Size	1/2 Recipe
Amount Per Serving	
Calories	**85**
	Kidney Friendly % DV*
Total Fat 0.5g	1%
Saturated Fat 0g	0%
Trans Fat 0g	
Cholesterol 0mg	0%
Total Carbohydrate 22g	8%
Dietary Fiber 2g	6%
Total Sugars 17g	
Includes 2g Added Sugar	4%
Protein 1g	
Sodium 0mg	0%
Potassium 240mg	7%
Phosphorus 25mg	2%
ORAC 3880	13%
Polyphenols 180mg	18%
AGE	VERY LOW
PRAL	-4.2
Dietary Nitrates	HIGH

*The % Daily Value (DV) tells you how much a nutrient in a serving of food contributes to the daily kidney friendly diet. 2,000 calories a day is used for general nutrition advice.

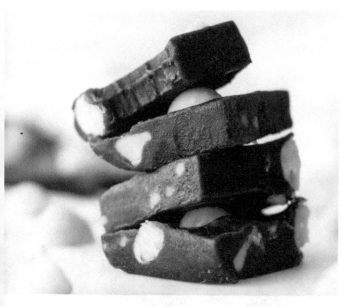

Macadamia Freezer Fudge

Prep Time: 15 minutes

Cook Time: 10 minutes

Serves 9

Healthy fudge? No, not really but pretty close. Freezer-friendly nut butters are used frequently in the raw food community. The idea here is to provide different taste and a calorie bomb. In the Paleo community, "Fat Bombs" are used to increase calories. Macadamia nuts are low in protein and high in healthy fats. You can get an extra 100 to 200 calories a day with this recipe, and it keeps well in the freezer. If your phosphorus levels are high, use carob powder instead of cocoa powder.

Ingredients:

½ cup (67 g) macadamia nuts, soaked for 2-4 hours and drained

3 tablespoons (45 ml) unsweetened rice milk (such as Rice Dream)

2 tablespoons (30 ml) coconut creamer (such as So Delicious)

3 tablespoons (42.6) real butter or smart balance

½ cup (62.5 g) calorie-free sweetener confectioners sugar(not granulated sugar)

2 tablespoons (14.76) cocoa or carob powder

½ teaspoon (2.6 g) pure vanilla extract

2 tablespoons (16.75 g) macadamia nuts, divided

Directions:

1. Combine the soaked and drained macadamia nuts, rice milk, and coconut creamer in a blender and process until very smooth. (You may need to stop the blender periodically to scrape the mixture from the sides.)

2. Combine the butter, confectioners sugar, and pureed macadamia mixture in a small saucepan over medium heat. Whisk constantly until mixture begins to bubble; reduce the heat to medium-low and continue stirring for 3-5 minutes, until the sauce is thickened and slightly browned. (As you are whisking, make sure to scrape down the sides of the saucepan so all of the mixture is continually heated and stirred.)

3. Remove the pan from the heat, and stir in the cocoa powder and vanilla extract. Pour the mixture into a small parchment paper-lined 2-quart square or rectangular dish. Press 1 tablespoon macadamia nuts into the fudge. Sprinkle the remaining nuts on top of the fudge.

4. Freeze the fudge for 2-3 hours, then score the fudge using a knife. Return to the freezer for an additional 2-3 hours before cutting. Store the fudge in the freezer for best results.

Nutrition Facts	
Serving Size	1/9 Recipe
Amount Per Serving	
Calories	**115**
	Kidney Friendly % DV*
Total Fat 6g	7%
Saturated Fat 1g	5%
Trans Fat 0g	
Cholesterol 0mg	0%
Total Carbohydrate 3g	1%
Dietary Fiber 0g	0%
Total Sugars 2g	
Includes 1g Added Sugar	2%
Protein 0g	
Sodium 35mg	2%
Potassium 195mg	4%
Phosphorus 15mg	1%
ORAC 950	3%
Polyphenols 95mg	9%
AGE	VERY LOW
PRAL	-3.6
Dietary Nitrates	LOW

* The % Daily Value (DV) tells you how much a nutrient in a serving of food contributes to the daily kidney friendly diet. 2,000 calories a day is used for general nutrition advice.

Cost Analysis:

Macadamia nuts are expensive, and it's hard to find unsalted nuts. Roasting is fine, but the salt is off limits. Amazon is a good source. Costs can run anywhere from $15.00 to $25.00 per pound. This recipe will cost around $5.00 to $6.00 for nine servings or about $0.66 a serving (servings are small).

Pears in Wine Sauce

Prep Time: 10 minutes

Cook Time: 30 minutes

Serves 1

This is a great dessert to serve when you have guests. Any extra wine sauce can be saved and will freeze well if you have cooked the alcohol out. This way you have it on-hand. The only real work is peeling the pears. They can be quartered or cut into smaller pieces if desired. You can also keep the pears whole if you like. Canned pears do not work as well since they are already full of water.

Ingredients:

5 tablespoons (7.5 g) calorie-free sweetener

¾ cup (180 ml) red wine

2 teaspoons (10 g) fresh lemon juice

1 teaspoon (5.3 g) pure vanilla extract

1 teaspoon (4 g) ground cinnamon

2 medium pears, peeled and cored

Directions:

1. Bring the sweetener, wine, lemon juice, vanilla and cinnamon to a boil in a small saucepan. Add the pears and cook over low heat for about 12 minutes or until soft.

2. Remove the pears and let the wine sauce simmer until reduced by half. Serve the pears with the wine sauce while still warm.

Cost Analysis:

With red wine at $1.00 and two pears at $2.00, this dessert is around $3.00 a serving.

Nutrition Facts	
Serving Size	Entire Recipe

Amount Per Serving	
Calories	**410**

	Kidney Friendly % DV*
Total Fat 0.5g	**1%**
Saturated Fat 0g	**0%**
Trans Fat 0g	
Cholesterol 0mg	**0%**
Total Carbohydrate 65g	**23%**
Dietary Fiber 5g	**17%**
Total Sugars 37g	
Includes 0g Added Sugar	**0%**
Protein 1g	

Sodium 10mg	1%
Potassium 690mg	20%
Phosphorus 85mg	7%
ORAC 19805	66%
Polyphenols 1170mg	117%
AGE	VERY LOW
PRAL	-13
Dietary Nitrates	HIGH

* The % Daily Value (DV) tells you how much a nutrient in a serving of food contributes to the daily kidney friendly diet. 2,000 calories a day is used for general nutrition advice.

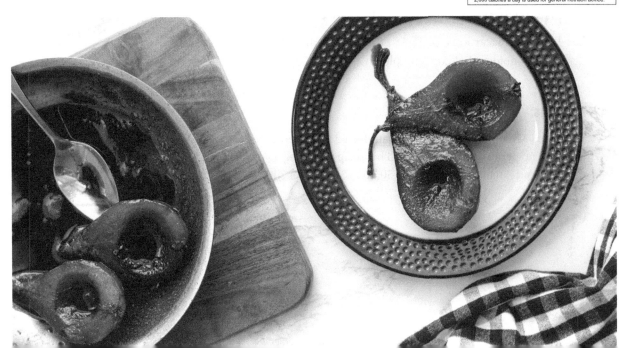

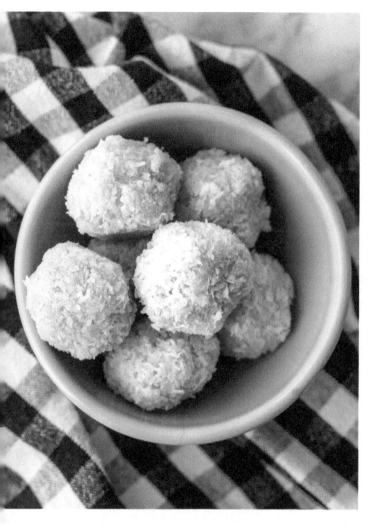

Coconut Macaroons

Prep Time: 15 minutes

Cook Time: 15 minutes

Serves 8

These cookies are so versatile. Change up the flavor profile by adding freeze-dried berries or carob chips. If you keep the cocoa powder to a dusting, you can also stir a little in for flavoring. Tapioca flour is available in most health oriented grocery stores, but it's also on Amazon. I was unable to find unsweetened and unsulphured shredded coconut in my local store, but Amazon has several brands. Bob's Red Mill brand is available online and in many stores.

Ingredients:

¾ cup (45 g) shredded unsweetened and unsulphured coconut

2 tablespoon (15.25 g)s tapioca flour or starch

2 tablespoons (40 g) pure maple syrup or sugar-free syrup substitute

½ teaspoon (2.6 g) pure vanilla extract

1 tablespoon (15 ml) unsweetened coconut milk (or other dairy-free milk)

Directions:

1. Preheat the oven to 300°F. Combine all of the ingredients in a small bowl. Mix together with a spoon, and then with your hands to press everything together. Shape mixture into 8 small balls, and place on a parchment paper-lined sheet pan.

2. Bake the macaroons for 15-18 minutes or until the undersides are slightly golden. Let cool completely.

Cost Analysis:

Bob's Red Mill unsweetened and unsulphured shredded coconut is about $0.66 per ounce on Amazon. This recipe calls for 45 grams (or 1.5 ounces), and it makes 8 servings so $0.20 to $0.25 a serving.

Nutrition Facts		
Serving Size		1/8 Recipe
Amount Per Serving		
Calories		**60**
		Kidney Friendly % DV*
Total Fat 4g		5%
Saturated Fat 4g		19%
Trans Fat 0g		
Cholesterol 0mg		0%
Total Carbohydrate 7g		2%
Dietary Fiber 1g		3%
Total Sugars 3g		
Includes 2g Added Sugar		6%
Protein 0g		
Sodium 0mg		0%
Potassium 35mg		1%
Phosphorus 10mg		1%
ORAC 15		0%
Polyphenols 5mg		1%
AGE		LOW
PRAL		-0.4
Dietary Nitrates		VERY LOW

* The % Daily Value (DV) tells you how much a nutrient in a serving of food contributes to the daily kidney friendly diet. 2,000 calories a day is used for general nutrition advice.

Raspberry Fool

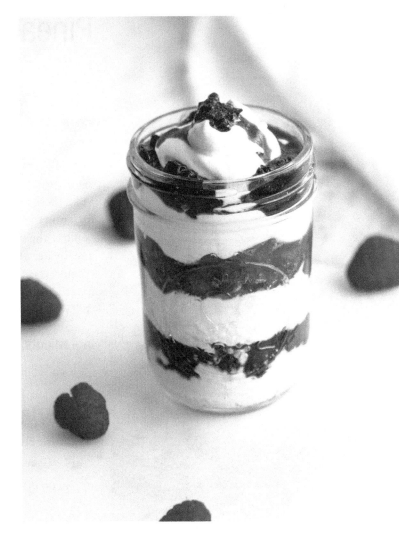

Prep Time: 15 minutes

Cook Time: 15 minutes

Serves 2

A fool is a British dessert combining fruit with custard, and this version takes only minutes to make. Be sure to use a whipped cream that is corn syrup free. (Do not use Cool Whip.) Cocowhip and Truwhip are in most grocery stores these days. You can use any low-potassium fruit in this dessert. Blackberries, strawberries, and blueberries are all great options. These days we just use fresh fruit and fresh berries. You don't have to cook the fruit if you don't want to.

Ingredients:

2 cups (200 g) raspberries (or use blackberries or blueberries)

1 tablespoon (15 g) fresh lemon juice, divided

2 tablespoons (15.6 g) calorie-free sweetener, divided (if needed)

1 tablespoon (15 ml) water

½ cup (37.5 g) cocowhip (such as So Delicious or Truwhip)

Directions:

1. Combine the raspberries, ½ tablespoon lemon juice, 1 tablespoon sweetener, and 1 tablespoon water in a small saucepan over medium-low heat. Cook, stirring frequently, until the berries begin to break down and the sauce thickens slightly. Remove the mixture from the saucepan and set aside.

2. Refrigerate and let cool for 20 to 30 minutes.

3. Layer the berry mixture with the cocowhip. Refrigerate the combined berries and whipped cream for at least 30 minutes before serving for the best results.

Cost Analysis:

The cost for Cocowhip and Truwhip is around $2.89 at my local store but can run as high as $3.89. We can say around $1.50 for the whipped cream and another $2.00 for the berries, equaling around $1.00 per serving.

Nutrition Facts		
Serving Size		1/2 Recipe
Amount Per Serving		
Calories		**110**
		Kidney Friendly % DV*
Total Fat 4g		6%
Saturated Fat 3g		15%
Trans Fat 0g		
Cholesterol 0mg		0%
Total Carbohydrate 20g		7%
Dietary Fiber 5g		18%
Total Sugars 10g		
Includes 5g Added Sugar		10%
Protein 1g		
Sodium 0mg		0%
Potassium 170mg		5%
Phosphorus 20mg		2%
ORAC 19310		64%
Polyphenols 580mg		58%
AGE		VERY LOW
PRAL		-3
Dietary Nitrates		HIGH

* The % Daily Value (DV) tells you how much a nutrient in a serving of food contributes to the daily kidney friendly diet. 2,000 calories a day is used for general nutrition advice.

Pineapple with Rum Sauce

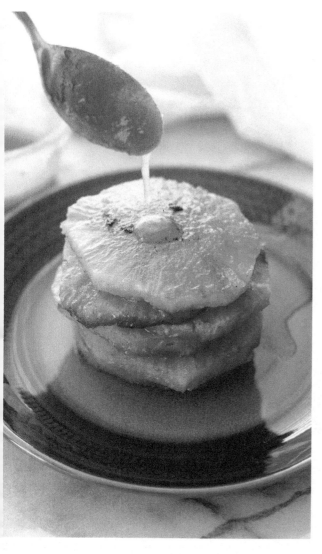

Prep Time: 10 minutes

Cook Time: 20 minutes

Serves 4

I had pineapples with rum some time ago, and we decided to try it again. Rum and wine desserts feel more decadent to me, so naturally I like these recipes. Pineapples are high in bromelain which reduces inflammation. Most of the alcohol is cooked out. Use more rum if you like the taste; the rum taste in this recipe is barely noticeable. For a really decadent dessert, spoon the pineapple with the sauce over ice cream. (Use the ice cream recipe in this chapter.) Or make pineapple ice cream and pour the rum sauce over the top. If you like to entertain this version will get rave reviews.

Ingredients:

1 cored pineapple, cut into ½-inch-thick rounds

1 teaspoon (4.7 g) melted butter (or use neutral oil)

1 tablespoon (12.9 g) brown sugar calorie-free sweetener like Splenda brown sugar

¼ cup (51.6 g) calorie-free sweetener

3 tablespoons (45 ml) water

2 tablespoons (30 ml) rum(can use white or dark rum, but dark is better)

½ teaspoon (2.6 g) pure vanilla extract

1 (3-inch) cinnamon stick

Nutrition Facts	
Serving Size	1/8 Recipe
Amount Per Serving	
Calories	**60**
	Kidney Friendly % DV*
Total Fat 4g	**5%**
Saturated Fat 4g	**19%**
Trans Fat 0g	
Cholesterol 0mg	**0%**
Total Carbohydrate 7g	**2%**
Dietary Fiber 1g	**3%**
Total Sugars 3g	
Includes 2g Added Sugar	**6%**
Protein 0g	
Sodium 0mg	0%
Potassium 35mg	1%
Phosphorus 10mg	1%
ORAC 15	0%
Polyphenols 5mg	1%
AGE	LOW
PRAL	-0.4
Dietary Nitrates	VERY LOW

* The % Daily Value (DV) tells you how much a nutrient in a serving of food contributes to the daily kidney friendly diet. 2,000 calories a day is used for general nutrition advice.

Directions:

1. Preheat the oven to 400°F. Toss the pineapple slices with butter or oil and brown sugar sweetener. Arrange on a parchment paper-lined sheet pan and bake for 15 minutes.

2. While the pineapple bakes, heat the sweetener, 3 tablespoons water, rum, vanilla, and cinnamon stick in a saucepan over medium heat. Cook until all of the sweetener is dissolved and the sauce begins to bubble.

3. Remove the pineapple from the oven. Increase the oven temperature to broil (max of 500°F). Carefully watch the slices as the parchment can burn at or above 500°F. Turn the pineapple slices over. Pour half of the sauce on top of the pineapple and spread evenly. Broil the pineapple until the tops are golden. Remove the pineapple from the oven, and serve with the remaining sauce.

Cost Analysis:

Pineapples cost about $3.00 each. This recipe includes about $0.50 worth of Splenda and sweetener. The rum cost should be tiny as well. Let's call this one $1.00 per serving.

Fresh Fruit with Vanilla Syrup

Prep Time: 5 minutes

Cook Time: 5 minutes

Serves 2

You can use almost any fruit here as long as you are watching the potassium and protein content. Mango is used to increase the diversity a little, and frozen/fresh mangos are easy to find. Fresh fruit by itself is great, but sometimes you'll want a change.

Ingredients:

¾ teaspoon (3.9 g) pure vanilla extract

3 to 4 tablespoons (45 ml) water

3 to 4 tablespoons (38.7 g) calorie-free sweetener

¾ cup (105 g) chopped mango

¾ cup (75 g) blueberries

½ pound (226.8 g) strawberries, halved or quartered

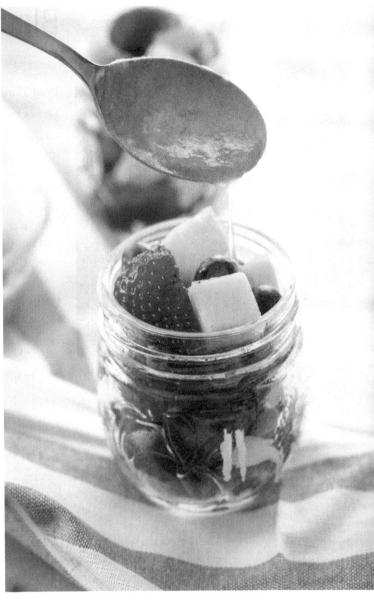

Directions:

1. Combine vanilla extract, water, and sweetener in a small saucepan over medium heat. Cook for a few minutes until the sweetener dissolves and the sauce begins to bubble.

2. Arrange the fruit in bowls or jars. Pour the syrup over the fruit. (If the syrup becomes too hard, place in a saucepan over low heat or heat in the microwave in 10-second increments.

Cost Analysis:

The cost for fruit will depend on the combination you choose and will run between $3.00 and $4.00 for two servings or around $2.00 per serving.

Nutrition Facts	
Serving Size	1/2 Recipe
Amount Per Serving	
Calories	**110**
	Kidney Friendly % DV*
Total Fat 0.5g	**1%**
Saturated Fat 0g	**0%**
Trans Fat 0g	
Cholesterol 0mg	**0%**
Total Carbohydrate 26g	**9%**
Dietary Fiber 4g	**14%**
Total Sugars 20g	
Includes 2g Added Sugar	**5%**
Protein 1g	
Sodium 0mg	0%
Potassium 290mg	8%
Phosphorus 40mg	3%
ORAC 9190	31%
Polyphenols 490mg	49%
AGE	VERY LOW
PRAL	-4.9
Dietary Nitrates	HIGH

* The % Daily Value (DV) tells you how much a nutrient in a serving of food contributes to the daily kidney friendly diet. 2,000 calories a day is used for general nutrition advice.

Blackberry Sangria Granita

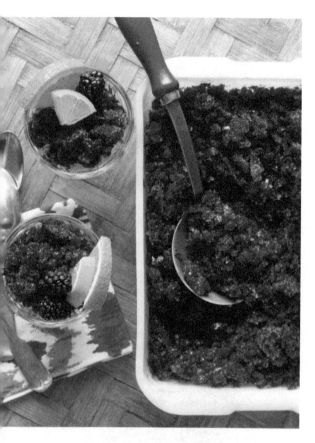

Prep Time: 20 minutes (not including freeze time)

Serves 8

Granita is a lightly frozen dessert, but if you are not careful it can turn into an iceberg. The alcohol helps keep the granita from turning into one chunk of ice. Polyphenols in blackberry and red wine make this another guilt-free dessert. The amount of alcohol per serving is very small. You can also freeze this recipe ice cube trays and add to sparkling water. Go easy on the wine if you go this route or the ice cube will not freeze all the way. If you ever needed an excuse to buy cheap wine, this is it.

Ingredients:

3 cups (432 g) fresh or frozen blackberries

¼ cup (12 g) calorie-free sweetener (such as Splenda)

1 cup (250 ml) water

1 tablespoon fresh lime juice

Juice and zest of 1 orange

1½ cups (360 ml) red wine

Garnish: fresh blackberries, orange wedges, lime wedges

Directions:

1. Mash blackberries and sweetener, and place in a strainer over a measuring cup or bowl. Strain, mashing the mixture with the back of a spoon.

2. Stir in water, lime juice, orange juice and zest, and red wine. Pour into a 9-inch baking dish. Freeze 8 hours or until firm.

3. Scrape with a fork into fluffy ice crystals. Serve in bowls with blackberries, orange wedges, and lime wedges, if desired.

Cost Analysis:

Wine and blackberries will normally cost about $8.00 to $10.00 combined. The recipe will average around $1.00 per serving.

Nutrition Facts

Serving Size	1/8 Recipe

Amount Per Serving

Calories	70

	Kidney Friendly % DV*
Total Fat 0g	0%
Saturated Fat 0g	0%
Trans Fat 0g	
Cholesterol 0mg	0%
Total Carbohydrate 9g	3%
Dietary Fiber 0g	0%
Total Sugars 4g	
Includes 1g Added Sugar	2%
Protein 1g	

Sodium 0mg	0%
Potassium 155mg	4%
Phosphorus 25mg	2%
ORAC 21055	40%
Polyphenols 410mg	41%
AGE	VERY LOW
PRAL	-2.7
Dietary Nitrates	HIGH

* The % Daily Value (DV) tells you how much a nutrient in a serving of food contributes to the daily kidney friendly diet. 2,000 calories a day is used for general nutrition advice.

Cherry Lemonade

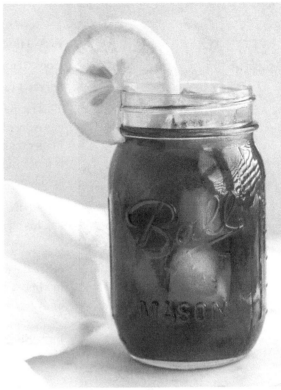

Prep Time: 10 minutes

Serves 1

Tart cherry is hard to use in any recipe. It's tart just like the name sounds. You could take a shot or few spoonfuls or add it to lemonade. The ORAC value is somewhere between 2,000 and 7,000 depending on the study you read and if a concentrate is used versus fresh juice. Tart cherry juice has been shown to reduce inflammation. I will keep saying this because we want as much diversity as we can get in our diet. This is another way to add some diversity. It's also great in the summertime.

Ingredients:

Ice cubes

¼ cup (60 ml) tart cherry juice

1 cup (250 ml) seltzer water (or water)

1½ tablespoons (22.5 g) fresh lemon juice

Calorie-free sweetener to taste

Directions:

Fill glass with ice cubes. Add remaining ingredients and stir to combine.

Cost Analysis:

Lemon are cheap, but tart cherry juice is not. Juice (not concentrate) will run between $0.15 and $0.25 an ounce. Concentrated (evaporated) juice is much more expensive, running just under a $1.00 per ounce in most cases. This recipe calls for two ounces of juice (not concentrate), so $0.50 a serving is a pretty good estimate.

Nutrition Facts

1 servings per recipe
Serving Size   1 1/4 Cup (10oz)

Amount Per Serving

Calories   40

	Kidney Friendly % DV*
Total Fat 0g	**0%**
Saturated Fat 0g	0%
Trans Fat 0g	
Cholesterol 0mg	**0%**
Total Carbohydrate 11g	**3%**
Dietary Fiber 0g	0%
Total Sugars 9g	
Includes 0g Added Sugar	0%
Protein 0g	
Sodium 35mg	2%
Potassium 100mg	2%
Phosphorus 95mg	8%
ORAC 2675	8%
Polyphenols 135mg	20%
AGE	VERY LOW
PRAL	1.3
Dietary Nitrates	MEDIUM

* The % Daily Value (DV) tells you how much a nutrient in a serving of food contributes to the daily kidney friendly diet. 2,000 calories a day is used for general nutrition advice.

Other kidney-friendly drinks:

- Apple Juice
- Latte/coffee espresso
- Black tea
- Chai Tea
- Cranberry Juice
- Iced or hot teas this includes herbal teas
- Water
- Cranberry juice
- Sparkling water
- Mineral water
- Beer *
- Wine*
- Arnold Palmer

Hibiscus Tea

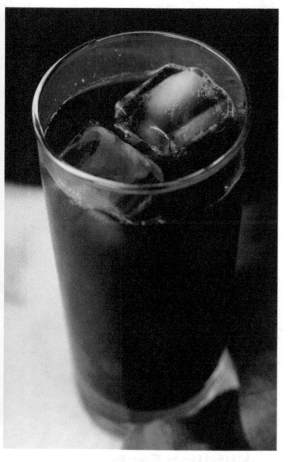

Prep Time: 20 minutes

Cook Time: 15 minutes

Serves 4 to 5

This recipe is for hibiscus tea concentrate. Why hibiscus you might ask? Hibiscus is very high in antioxidants, 6,900 on the ORAC scale. This is 2 to 3 times higher than coffee or black tea. Everyone thinks green tea is king, but hibiscus is much higher (with the exception of Matcha powder). Two glasses of hot or cold hibiscus tea get you almost halfway to your antioxidant goal for the day.

My advice is to brew the tea as strong and drink as strong as you can stand it. This advice holds true for all teas and coffees

Stay away from traditional bagged teas if you can. Many are mixed with other flavors or herbs to reduce costs and this waters down the ORAC value in almost all cases. You can buy a one pound bag of organic hibiscus leaves on Amazon for $12.00. One pound will last a very long time.

Ingredients:

¾ cup (24 g) dried hibiscus leaves

1½ (375 ml) cups water

Sugar substitute (such as Splenda or stevia)

Directions:

1. Combine the hibiscus leaves and water In a small saucepan. Bring to a boil; stir, and reduce the heat to low. Simmer about 12 minutes.

2. Remove the saucepan from the heat. Pour the liquid into a strainer over a liquid measuring cup, gently pressing the leaves into the strainer.

3. For each cup of hibiscus tea, combine about ¼ cup of the concentrate with ¼ - ½ cup hot water. Sweeten to taste.

Nutrition Facts

4 servings per recipe

Serving Size   1 1/2 Cup (12oz)

Amount Per Serving

Calories   **0**

	Kidney Friendly % DV*
Total Fat 0g	0%
Saturated Fat 0g	0%
Trans Fat 0g	
Cholesterol 0mg	0%
Total Carbohydrate 0g	0%
Dietary Fiber 0g	0%
Total Sugars 0g	
Includes 0g Added Sugar	0%
Protein 0g	
Sodium 10mg	0%
Potassium 50mg	0%
Phosphorus 0mg	0%
ORAC 1750	6%
Polyphenols 45mg	4%
AGE	VERY LOW
PRAL	-0.3
Dietary Nitrates	MEDIUM

* The % Daily Value (DV) tells you how much a nutrient in a serving of food contributes to the daily kidney friendly diet. 2,000 calories a day is used for general nutrition advice.

Cost Analysis:

Buying a bulk bag of hibiscus leaves will yield a cost per cup of between $0.25 and $0.50 per large glass.

Note about teas:

Teas are the most cost effective option for adding antioxidants to your diet. Consuming two or three glasses of teas can add anywhere from 5,000 to 17,000 ORAC units a day. In most cases the cost of homemade tea is less than 50 cents. Consuming a few cups or glasses of teas each day allow you to be a little more relaxed with your diet as well. Converting to a latte or adding a milk substitute adds calories. Your antioxidant levels decline in a few hours after each meal, so teas keep adding antioxidants between meals.

If you are on a tight budget, teas can make your antioxidant dollars go a long way.

Blackberry Iced Tea

Prep Time: 5 minutes (not including cool time)

Cook Time: 10 minutes

Serves 4

Adding blackberries to iced tea is great tasting and increases antioxidants/polyphenols totals. As you can see, we are always trying to increase nutrition when we can.

Ingredients:

2 cups (288 g) fresh or frozen blackberries (plus more for garnish)

2 tablespoons (3 g) calorie-free sweetener (such as Splenda)

3 black tea bags

4 cups (1 L) water

Ice cubes

Lemon wedges, mint sprigs

Additional sweetener, if desired

Directions:

1. Mash blackberries and sweetener in a bowl with a potato masher or fork.

2. Boil water and add tea bags. Let stand and steep 8 minutes. Discard bags.

3. Pour tea over blackberry mixture. Let cool, and strain. Serve over ice cubes and garnish with additional blackberries, lemon wedges, and mint sprigs, if desired.

Cost Analysis:

This is less than $0.50 per serving.

Nutrition Facts	
Serving Size	1/4 Recipe
Amount Per Serving	
Calories	**35**
	Kidney Friendly % DV*
Total Fat 0g	0%
Saturated Fat 0g	0%
Trans Fat 0g	
Cholesterol 0mg	0%
Total Carbohydrate 9g	3%
Dietary Fiber 0g	0%
Total Sugars 5g	
Includes 1g Added Sugar	2%
Protein 1g	
Sodium 0mg	0%
Potassium 120mg	3%
Phosphorus 15mg	1%
ORAC 14150	47%
Polyphenols 410mg	41%
AGE	VERY LOW
PRAL	-2.1
Dietary Nitrates	VERY HIGH

* The % Daily Value (DV) tells you how much a nutrient in a serving of food contributes to the daily kidney friendly diet. 2,000 calories a day is used for general nutrition advice.

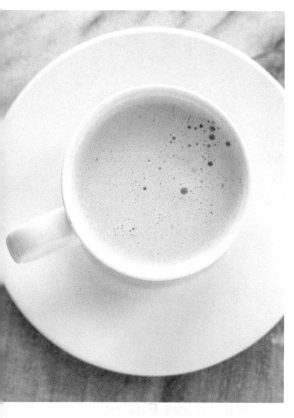

Matcha Latte

Prep Time: 10 minutes

Cook Time: 5 minutes (for hot latte)

Serves 1

Green tea is great for you as well. Matcha is a green tea ground into a fine powder. This powder is consumed with the tea. This is something a little new to most of us. By consuming the actual tea leaves vs the powder, the antioxidant value may be increased by 100 times versus traditional bagged or infused teas. Adding a plant based milk increases the calories if needed, You can enjoy this drink either hot or cold. If you have an immersion blender or milk frother, use it in step 2 in place of a whisk to yield a frothier latte. For an iced latte, consider adding a small amount (¼ teaspoon) of additional matcha since the ice cubes will dilute the latte.

Some form of Matcha is available in most grocery stores (but not all). Do not buy the premade latte versions. You will read online about people speaking about Matcha much like wine Amazon has a wide variety as well. One more note: White tea matcha powder is the same leaf as the green tea. White tea is a little harder to find, but has less of a grassy taste.

Ingredients:

¾ cup plus 2 tablespoons (206.56 ml) unsweetened rice milk (such as Rice Dream)

¼ cup coconut creamer (60 ml) (such as So Delicious)

1 teaspoon (1.5 g) matcha powder

Calorie-free sweetener (such as Splenda or stevia), optional

Directions:

For a hot latte:

1. Combine the rice milk and coconut creamer in a small saucepan over medium heat and simmer until hot. (Or microwave on HIGH at 30-second intervals until the mixture reaches desired thickness.)

2. Spoon the matcha powder into a mug. Slowly add the rice milk mixture, whisking until combined. Sweeten with sugar substitute, if desired.

For an iced latte:

1. Combine all ingredients together in a blender and process until well combined.

2. Pour over ice and serve.

Cost Analysis:

On Amazon, the best selling Matcha powders are running $0.33 to $0.40 per serving. Or, around $10.00 for a 30-gram bag.

Nutrition Facts	
1 servings per recipe	
Serving Size	**1 Cup (8oz)**
Amount Per Serving	
Calories	**150**
	Kidney Friendly % DV*
Total Fat 4g	5%
Saturated Fat 2g	10%
Trans Fat 0g	
Cholesterol 0mg	0%
Total Carbohydrate 22g	8%
Dietary Fiber 0g	0%
Total Sugars 10g	
Includes 0g Added Sugar	0%
Protein 2g	
Sodium 85mg	4%
Potassium 65mg	2%
Phosphorus 55mg	5%
ORAC 25	0%
Polyphenols 0mg	0%
AGE	LOW
PRAL	0.5
Dietary Nitrates	LOW

* The % Daily Value (DV) tells you how much a nutrient in a serving of food contributes to the daily kidney friendly diet. 2,000 calories a day is used for general nutrition advice.

Fruit and Trail Mix

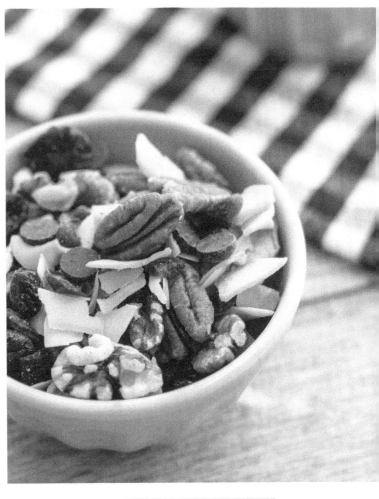

Prep Time: 5 minutes

Serves 4

Trail mix is a tough one, but I wanted to have something to snack on based on a few emails. This recipe is pretty good, but remember you have to track the protein and potassium. You can also used spiced or sweetened pecans if you like.

Ingredients:

½ cup apple chips, torn into pieces

¼ cup reduced-sugar dried cranberries

¼ cup macadamia nuts

¼ cup pecans

¼ dried pineapple (unsweetened if you can find it)

2 tablespoons carob chips (optional)

Directions:

Toss together all ingredients in a large bowl and enjoy!

Cost Analysis:

The nuts increase the costs to around $1.00 to $1.25 per serving.

Other kidney-friendly snacks:

- Smart pop/Air Popped popcorn
- Pecans/Macadamia nuts in moderation
- Fresh or frozen Apples, pears, raspberries, blackberries
- Dried fruit, apples, cranberries, pears in moderation
- Taste connection bread mixes

Nutrition Facts

4 servings per recipe

Serving Size	56g

Amount Per Serving	
Calories	**240**

	Kidney Friendly % DV*
Total Fat 13g	**16%**
Saturated Fat 3g	**15%**
Trans Fat 0g	
Cholesterol 0mg	**0%**
Total Carbohydrate 33g	**12%**
Dietary Fiber 4g	**13%**
Total Sugars 23g	
Includes 2g Added Sugar	**4%**
Protein 2g	
Sodium 5mg	0%
Potassium 135mg	4%
Phosphorus 40mg	3%
ORAC 3270	11%
Polyphenols 270mg	27%
AGE	LOW
PRAL	-1.5
Dietary Nitrates	LOW

* The % Daily Value (DV) tells you how much a nutrient in a serving of food contributes to the daily kidney friendly diet. 2,000 calories a day is used for general nutrition advice.

Milk Substitute

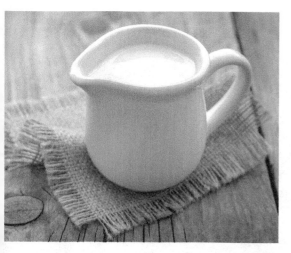

I really wanted a clever name for this because it's so close it will fool most people. The taste is a little different, but close enough you likely wouldn't.

"Filk" for fake milk was the only name I could come up, but who wants to drink something called filk. Anyway, this recipe can be used whenever milk is needed or if you would like a glass of milk. If you have a better name, please email me.

The sheer number of milk substitutes has dramatically increased over the past ten years. Almond, soy, rice, hazelnut, oat, coconut, and hemp, to name a few. This makes finding a suitable substitute much easier. MAKE SURE TO READ ALL LABELS before using any of these plant-based substitutes. Many have added phosphorus and potassium.

We will use Rice Dream (or other brand) of unenriched (also called original) rice milk. Do not use the enriched version. The enriched version contains added phosphorus which we don't want. Remember, phosphorus as a food additive is absorbed by 80% + by our bodies. Plant-based phosphorus is absorbed at half this rate.

The other ingredient is coconut creamer. The "So Delicious" brand of coconut milk creamer is available in almost all grocery store these days. The downside is the cost, and it contains some amount of dipotassium phosphate, aka phosphorus. This is one of the last ingredients on the label and we use a smaller amount, so it's a trade-off. I have contacted So Delicious several times, but no one has been able to tell me the exact amount of dipotassium phosphate. In the future, I would like to test all of the plant-based milks to determine exactly what is in each version, but that will have to wait for now. The amount is likely very small and we don't use a large amount, so I think it's an okay trade-off.

Coconut creamer provides an extra 100 to 120 calories with no protein, so this is a big help. However, due to additives, I would keep this to two cups a day or less.

One more bit of data: since this isn't cow's milk, you can't expect to get the same results if you use this in a traditional recipe.

Filk is great for the following:

- Use for coffee, tea, lattes, and Chai's
- Use in soup recipes instead of creamer or milk
- Drink as a milk substitute
- Use in smoothies or blended drinks

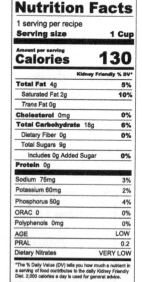

Nutrition Facts		
1 serving per recipe		
Serving size		**1 Cup**
Amount per serving		
Calories		**130**
		Kidney Friendly % DV*
Total Fat 4g		5%
Saturated Fat 2g		10%
Trans Fat 0g		
Cholesterol 0mg		0%
Total Carbohydrate 18g		6%
Dietary Fiber 0g		0%
Total Sugars 9g		
Includes 0g Added Sugar		0%
Protein 0g		
Sodium 75mg		3%
Potassium 60mg		2%
Phosphorus 50g		4%
ORAC 0		0%
Polyphenols 0mg		0%
AGE		LOW
PRAL		0.2
Dietary Nitrates		VERY LOW
*The % Daily Value (DV) tells you how much a nutrient in a serving of food contributes to the daily Kidney Friendly Diet. 2,000 calories a day is used for general advice.		

If you like it, the best practice is to use a small pitcher and mix it together and leave it in the refrigerator to use as needed. Remember to shake before using. You can fine-tune this recipe to your liking, but it's pretty good as is.

Your feedback on any recipes is always appreciated and much needed to help me improve the diet and treatment program.

The basic recipe for one cup is:

- ¾ cup Unenriched rice milk
- ¼ cup So Delicious Coconut milk creamer

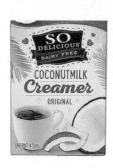

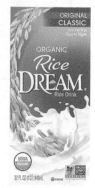

The price for Rice Dream "original"is generally $3.19 for a 32 oz box at my local store. Coconut milk creamer is $2.19 for a small 16 oz carton. Cost per cup mixed together is around 10 to 11 cents per oz or 80 cents for an 8 oz cup. This makes it significantly cheaper than bottled water or soft drinks.

DRINK NUTRITION

Apple Juice

Nutrition Facts

Serving Size 1 Cup (8oz)

Amount Per Serving

Calories 115

Kidney Friendly % DV*

Total Fat 0g	0%
Saturated Fat 0g	0%
Trans Fat 0g	
Cholesterol 0mg	0%
Total Carbohydrate 28g	10%
Dietary Fiber 0g	0%
Total Sugars 24g	
Includes 0g Added Sugar	0%
Protein 0g	
Sodium 10mg	0%
Potassium 250mg	7%
Phosphorus 15mg	1%
ORAC 1035	3%
Polyphenols 355mg	35%
AGE	VERY LOW
PRAL	-2.2
Dietary Nitrates	LOW

* The % Daily Value (DV) tells you how much a nutrient in a serving of food contributes to the daily kidney friendly diet. 2,000 calories a day is used for general nutrition advice.

Arnold Palmer

Nutrition Facts

Serving Size 1 Cup (8oz)

Amount Per Serving

Calories 70

Kidney Friendly % DV*

Total Fat 0g	0%
Saturated Fat 0g	0%
Trans Fat 0g	
Cholesterol 0mg	0%
Total Carbohydrate 17g	6%
Dietary Fiber 0g	0%
Total Sugars 17g	
Includes 15g Added Sugar	30%
Protein 0g	
Sodium 0mg	0%
Potassium 65mg	5%
Phosphorus 0mg	0%
ORAC 1045	3%
Polyphenols 125mg	12%
AGE	VERY LOW
PRAL	-0.6
Dietary Nitrates	LOW

* The % Daily Value (DV) tells you how much a nutrient in a serving of food contributes to the daily kidney friendly diet. 2,000 calories a day is used for general nutrition advice.

Black Tea

Nutrition Facts

Serving Size 1 Cup (8oz)

Amount Per Serving

Calories 0

Kidney Friendly % DV*

Total Fat 0g	0%
Saturated Fat 0g	0%
Trans Fat 0g	
Cholesterol 0mg	0%
Total Carbohydrate 0g	0%
Dietary Fiber 0g	0%
Total Sugars 0g	
Includes 0g Added Sugar	0%
Protein 0g	
Sodium 5mg	0%
Potassium 90mg	3%
Phosphorus 0mg	0%
ORAC 1690	6%
Polyphenols 255mg	25%
AGE	VERY LOW
PRAL	-0.3
Dietary Nitrates	LOW

* The % Daily Value (DV) tells you how much a nutrient in a serving of food contributes to the daily kidney friendly diet. 2,000 calories a day is used for general nutrition advice.

Chai Tea

Nutrition Facts

Serving Size 1 Cup (8oz)

Amount Per Serving

Calories 0

Kidney Friendly % DV*

Total Fat 0g	0%
Saturated Fat 0g	0%
Trans Fat 0g	
Cholesterol 0mg	0%
Total Carbohydrate 0g	0%
Dietary Fiber 0g	0%
Total Sugars 0g	
Includes 0g Added Sugar	0%
Protein 0g	
Sodium 5mg	0%
Potassium 0mg	0%
Phosphorus 0mg	0%
ORAC 2555	9%
Polyphenols 125mg	12%
AGE	VERY LOW
PRAL	-0.3
Dietary Nitrates	LOW

* The % Daily Value (DV) tells you how much a nutrient in a serving of food contributes to the daily kidney friendly diet. 2,000 calories a day is used for general nutrition advice.

Coffee

Nutrition Facts

Serving Size 1 Cup (8oz)

Amount Per Serving

Calories 5

Kidney Friendly % DV*

Total Fat 0g	0%
Saturated Fat 0g	0%
Trans Fat 0g	
Cholesterol 0mg	0%
Total Carbohydrate 0g	0%
Dietary Fiber 0g	0%
Total Sugars 0g	
Includes 0g Added Sugar	0%
Protein 0g	
Sodium 5mg	0%
Potassium 116mg	3%
Phosphorus 10mg	0%
ORAC 6725	22%
Polyphenols 920mg	92%
AGE	VERY LOW
PRAL	-1.4
Dietary Nitrates	LOW

* The % Daily Value (DV) tells you how much a nutrient in a serving of food contributes to the daily kidney friendly diet. 2,000 calories a day is used for general nutrition advice.

Cranberry Juice

Nutrition Facts

Serving Size 1 Cup (8oz)

Amount Per Serving

Calories 115

Kidney Friendly % DV*

Total Fat 0g	0%
Saturated Fat 0g	0%
Trans Fat 0g	
Cholesterol 0mg	0%
Total Carbohydrate 30g	11%
Dietary Fiber 0g	0%
Total Sugars 30g	
Includes 0g Added Sugar	0%
Protein 0g	
Sodium 5mg	0%
Potassium 195mg	5%
Phosphorus 35mg	3%
ORAC 3630	12%
Polyphenols 140mg	14%
AGE	VERY LOW
PRAL	-3.0
Dietary Nitrates	LOW

* The % Daily Value (DV) tells you how much a nutrient in a serving of food contributes to the daily kidney friendly diet. 2,000 calories a day is used for general nutrition advice.

Herbal Tea

Nutrition Facts

Serving Size 1 Cup (8oz)

Amount Per Serving

Calories 0

Kidney Friendly % DV*

Total Fat 0g	0%
Saturated Fat 0g	0%
Trans Fat 0g	
Cholesterol 0mg	0%
Total Carbohydrate 0g	0%
Dietary Fiber 0g	0%
Total Sugars 0g	
Includes 0g Added Sugar	0%
Protein 0g	
Sodium 0mg	0%
Potassium 0mg	0%
Phosphorus 0mg	0%
ORAC 17475	58%
Polyphenols 135mg	13%
AGE	VERY LOW
PRAL	-0.3
Dietary Nitrates	LOW

* The % Daily Value (DV) tells you how much a nutrient in a serving of food contributes to the daily kidney friendly diet. 2,000 calories a day is used for general nutrition advice.

Latte

Nutrition Facts

Serving Size 1 Cup (8oz)

Amount Per Serving

Calories 70

Kidney Friendly % DV*

Total Fat 3g	4%
Saturated Fat 1.5g	8%
Trans Fat 0g	
Cholesterol 10mg	3%
Total Carbohydrate 6g	2%
Dietary Fiber 0g	0%
Total Sugars 7g	
Includes 0g Added Sugar	0%
Protein 4g	
Sodium 65mg	3%
Potassium 275mg	8%
Phosphorus 120mg	10%
ORAC 4235	14%
Polyphenols 960mg	96%
AGE	LOW
PRAL	-1.2
Dietary Nitrates	LOW

* The % Daily Value (DV) tells you how much a nutrient in a serving of food contributes to the daily kidney friendly diet. 2,000 calories a day is used for general nutrition advice.

Red Wine

Nutrition Facts

Serving Size 1 Glass (5oz)

Amount Per Serving

Calories 120

Kidney Friendly % DV*

Total Fat 0g	0%
Saturated Fat 0g	0%
Trans Fat 0g	
Cholesterol 0mg	0%
Total Carbohydrate 4g	1%
Dietary Fiber 0g	0%
Total Sugars 1g	
Includes 0g Added Sugar	0%
Protein 0g	
Sodium 5mg	0%
Potassium 195mg	5%
Phosphorus 35mg	3%
ORAC 5625	19%
Polyphenols 335mg	33%
AGE	VERY LOW
PRAL	-2.4
Dietary Nitrates	HIGH

* The % Daily Value (DV) tells you how much a nutrient in a serving of food contributes to the daily kidney friendly diet. 2,000 calories a day is used for general nutrition advice.

Regular Beer

Nutrition Facts

Serving Size 1 Can (12oz)

Amount Per Serving

Calories 150

Kidney Friendly % DV*

Total Fat 0g	0%
Saturated Fat 0g	0%
Trans Fat 0g	
Cholesterol 0mg	0%
Total Carbohydrate 12g	4%
Dietary Fiber 0g	0%
Total Sugars 1g	
Includes 0g Added Sugar	0%
Protein 1g	
Sodium 15mg	0%
Potassium 95mg	3%
Phosphorus 50mg	4%
ORAC 400	2%
Polyphenols 75mg	7%
AGE	VERY LOW
PRAL	-0.2
Dietary Nitrates	VERY LOW

* The % Daily Value (DV) tells you how much a nutrient in a serving of food contributes to the daily kidney friendly diet. 2,000 calories a day is used for general nutrition advice.

MEAL PLANNING EXAMPLES

Planning your meals, calories, protein, etc. will determine your success or failure to a large degree. Plant-based diets without fried foods are normally very low in calories. It's very easy to start losing weight or feel hungry all of the time because a healthy plant-based diet will normally yield only 1,000 to 1,500 calories a day. We will be short of our 1,800 calorie goal on most days. This is where planning pays off big time.

It's easy to plan to hit a certain target number of calories each day, you just have to crunch the numbers and see if you are short or not.

If you have a calorie shortfall, you have lots of options. I say keep it simple by using a combination of the following:

Increase a serving size of a certain meal or dessert by 50%, 100%, or even 200% if needed

Add a snack or smoothie

Add fruit juice like cranberry juice

Add plant-based milk to coffee and teas

Simple and trackable is always better. If you try to adjust every meal or every snack you will go a little crazy. Adjust just one meal as needed for the day or add one or two simple snacks. Try to keep as many meals as simple as possible. This makes tracking calories and protein intake much easier. Don't make it complicated by adding something different to each meal.

We have prepared a few meal plans for you. These meals plan are educational in nature. Yes, you can follow them, but the main purpose is to show you what it looks like to plan and adjust each day. It takes just a few minutes to do each day - or better yet, plan the week in advance. You should understand that planning and adjusting calories are a daily thing for us.

Everyone will have to adjust based on their individual calorie needs or other restrictions. The key point is that a few minutes of planning means you won't be short on calories, start losing weight, or feel like you are starving all the time.

Expect to adjust each day as needed. I hope the examples help.

Sample Meal Planning

List shortfalls and suggested solutions if needed.

Each day will have different totals for each area, protein, calories, etc...

The average over a week or so is what matters. You can go a little over or a little under each day as long as your average intake is at the desired levels. If run high on everything one day, make sure you are low enough the next day to hit your numbers.

You will see several meals plans both above and the below the desired numbers. I wanted to show this fact as this is what happens in real life."

1,800 calorie target, max 30 grams of protein, 3,500 potassium

AMERICANA	Calories	Protein	Potassium	ORAC	Polyphenols	PRAL	Nitrates
Berry fool	110	1	170	19310	580	-3	High
Portobello with mashed potatoes or cauliflower	625	12	1765	6965	405	-21.8	Medium
beet salad	700	5	655	14140	910	-9.4	Very High
blabarssoppa	280	2	185	19255	445	-2.2	Very Low
Total Calories	**1715**	**20**	**2775**	**59670**	**2340**	**-9.4**	**Medium**
Shortfall	**-85**						
add snack of apple, fruit juice or 100 calorie snack	100	1	195	5020	350	-1.9	Low
New Total	**1815**	**21**	**2955**	**51050**	**2328**	**-9.2**	**Medium**

MEXICAN	Calories	Protein	Potassium	ORAC	Polyphenols	PRAL	Nitrates
Huevo ranchero	210	13	490	1870	210	-3.2	Low
Pumpkin soup with chorizo	275	6	735	15180	620	-7.9	Low
veggie fajitas with tostada salad	665	12	1825	16595	1190	-23.5	Medium
pineapple with rum	125	1	190	990	260	-3.9	Very Low
Total Calories	**1275**	**32**	**3240**	**34635**	**2280**	**-9.6**	**Low**
Shortfall	**-575**						
Apple	100	1	195	5020	350	-1.9	Low
2 cups blueberries	165	1	310	13835	830	-2.7	High
Cranberry juice 2 glasses	230	0	390	7260	1920	-3	Low
New Total	**1770**	**34**	**4135**	**60750**	**5380**	**-9.4**	**Medium**

ITALIAN	Calories	Protein	Potassium	ORAC	Polyphenols	PRAL	Nitrates
Polenta with berries	400	8	260	15955	1165	0.4	High
Sweet potato with side salads	295	4	665	3650	340	-11.7	Medium
Pesto with zucchini	510	3	475	2555	190	-7.3	Medium
Watermelon blueberry sorbet	85	1	240	3830	180	-4.2	High
Total Calories	**1290**	**16**	**1640**	**25990**	**1875**	**-5.9**	**Medium**
Shortfall	**-510**						
Double serving dinner of Pesto with Zuccuni	510	3	310	13835	830	-2.7	High
New Total	**1800**	**22**	**2425**	**42375**	**2895**	**-5.6**	**Medium**

FRENCH	Calories	Protein	Potassium	ORAC	Polyphenols	PRAL	Nitrates
Cinnamon apples	395	2	540	16470	1095	-9.1	Low
Main dish salad	305	3	525	3680	210	-9.4	High
Mushroom bourguignon	255	6	1190	6180	265	-15	Medium
Bread (2 large slices of Taste Essentials bread)	205	0	0	0	0	0	
Pears in wine sauce	410	1	690	19805	1170	-13	High
Total Calories	**1570**	**12**	**2945**	**46135**	**2740**	**-7.1**	**Medium**
Shortfall	**-230**						
Two cups of coffee with plant based creamer	140	2	185	2015	115	-0.2	Low
1 cup of cranberry juice	115	0	195	3630	960	-9.4	Low
New Total	1825	14	3325	51780	3815		

SPANISH	Calories	Protein	Potassium	ORAC	Polyphenols	PRAL	Nitrates
Shakshuka	200	11	770	1485	105	-9.1	Low
Tortilla soup with tortilla chips and salsa(what is serving of tortilla chips) - 30g is a serving of tortilla chips	520	8	640	24605	960	-7.1	Low
Tapas night-Peppers, Gazpacho, carrots	455	6	1050	3895	635	-6.2	Medium
Blackberry Sangria sorbet	70	1	155	21055	410	-2.7	High
Total Calories	**1245**	**26**	**2615**	**51040**	**2110**	**-6.9**	**Medium**
Shortfall	**-555**						
Two cups of a latte with plant based milk at breakfast	140	2	185	2015	115	-0.2	Low
Double blackberry sangria serving	140	3	465	63165	1230	-8.1	High
Extra serving of torilla chips and salsa with lunch	170	2	195	5020	350	-1.9	Low
1 cup of cranberry juice	115	0	195	3630	960	-9.4	Low
New Total	**1810**	**33**	**3460**	**121240**	**3805**	**-17.1**	

SOUTHERN	Calories	Protein	Potassium	ORAC	Polyphenols	PRAL	Nitrates
Fruit and pecan bowl	340	3	200	10815	630	-2.7	High
Corn and chili soup with collard greens	400	9	650	30150	710	-7.2	Medium
Jackfruit crab cakes with coleslaw	395	8	835	17035	175	-8.4	Low
Fresh fruit with vanilla syrup	105	1	285	9175	485	-4.9	High
New Total	**1240**	**21**	**1970**	**67175**	**2000**	**-5.8**	**Medium**
Shortfall	**-560**						
Double serving of Fresh Fruit with vanilla syrup	105	0	195	4235	960	-3	Low
Matcha Latte x 2	140	2	185	2015	115	-0.2	Low
Increase Jackfruit crabcakes and coleslaw serving size by 50%	342	5	200	850	490	2.1	Low
New Total	**1827**	**28**	**2550**	**74275**	**3565**	**-6.9**	**Medium**

SUMMARY

I consider this book version 1.0: the worst version of the book or our starting point towards a kickass recipe/meal book in the future. My goal is to have such a great diet that we can increase dietary compliance by a measurable amount. Low-cost, fun, and a little decadent is the idea.

Next year will be version 2.0 and so on. I hope to add and subtract from this book each year.

Your input is needed at www.stoppingkidneydisease.com/recipeinput to rate recipes. Please rate recipes you have tried. Please do not rate recipes if have not prepared and consumed the recipe. Just because a recipe is not appealing to you, you shouldn't assume it's a bad recipe. In order to get free recipes in the future, make sure you are on the list at www.stoppingkidneydisease.com.

Living well, living longer, and living better is possible with incurable kidney disease. You don't have to eat "grass" like several patients have commented and you don't have to starve or lose weight. The diet can be tasty and diverse despite the restrictions. You can eat decadent desserts, foods from all over the world, meals you can serve to family and friends, and eat cheaper than almost any alternative.

The food cost per day is between $9.00 and $15.00. The cost of an average fast food meal is around $7.00 One cup of coffee and one fast food meal will cost about the same as this diet. Cost is not a valid objection, in my opinion.

What about other valid objections? Are there any valid objections not to try the diet and treatment plan? Here are a few I have heard over the past year. I will let you decide.

Let's see:

I don't want to change what I eat

I don't like certain foods

I was told not to eat "X" food(s)

I can't give up " X " food

I don't like to cook

You don't understand, I have eaten "X" foods my whole life

I don't have the time

I don't like planning my meals and feeling like I have to eat "X" meals every day

I am going to wait and see what happens this year

… and the list goes on.

Are any of these really valid objections? Let's think about these objections vs. the outcome.

What's more important, not changing or maybe adding years to your life?

What's more important, not trying new things or maybe adding years to your life?

What's more important, continuing to eat a certain food or maybe adding years to your life?

… and so on.

These objections seem silly when you consider the consequences.

If your bloodwork is not getting better, you know it's time for a change anyway.

None of these make sense in real life or stand up to any kind of scrutiny. Think about it from another viewpoint:

What if you met a cancer patient who told you the following:

They have an incurable form of cancer and diet may be the only option to slowing or stopping the progression of cancer. The diet is no guarantee, but other cancer patients have had success with it. However, they didn't want to change what they are eating right now. They decided to "wait and see" what happens over the upcoming years.

What would your opinion be?

99.9% of us would say, "It's only a diet, they should at least try it to see if it works or not. They have nothing to lose".

Kidney diets are really no different if you think about it. Diets are hard, I will be the first to admit this after years of struggling. In fact, I still struggle after all these years. Dr. Walser's diet felt overwhelming to me at first. At Johns Hopkins, I was given a folder with some photocopied information and told "Good luck, see you in a month." This is not a complaint about Johns Hopkins, but a reminder that at the time, I knew less than zero about diets and how my kidneys worked. My experience at Johns Hopkins was life-changing, but I think we underestimate how little most of us actually know about nutrition, our kidneys, and our disease.

Looking back, very little guidance was given. The reasons are multiple, but the biggest reason (in my opinion) is we didn't know what we should be eating except for reducing protein. I don't want this to happen to you, which is why I have written this book. We all need as much support and education as possible.

Yes, special diets are hard, but the alternatives are much, much harder. Losing kidney function, getting more comorbid conditions each year, feeling worse, and your odds getting lower every year is a million times worse that sticking with a diet for 90 days to see if it will help you or not.

Education as a goal

My main goal is education. I have seen firsthand over the years that educated patients make better decisions. I also believe with 100% certainty that educated patients live longer and better lives. The more educated you are about your kidneys, disease, and treatment options, the better your odds. I think this is a law that will never be broken.

Patients start automatically making better choices after they get educated.

The reality of our situation is that "incurable" translates to "it's up to you to find an answer." It's up to you to get educated on your options. It's up to you to stay on a certain diet. It's up to you to seek out treatment options.

I hope this book educates you on the pitfalls and flaws of traditional kidney diets, so you can make better choices going forward. I also hope this book helps you improve your health, slow or stop your disease, and have a better quality of life than ever before.

Do yourself a favor: Give it 90 days and see what happens. You have nothing to lose and everything to gain. If you get good results after 90 days, then stick with it. You have a black and white answer if the diet works for you. You don't have to guess.

I know some of you view this change with hesitation, but there is nothing to fear. I promise you I am a "hard case." If a hard-headed guy from Texas/Louisiana who grew up raising cattle, worked as a cowboy in the summers, served in the military, and still dreams about Texas barbeque joints can make the change, then there is hope for all of us. This I promise. It took me 10 years to get educated and start making real progress after my diagnosis. If you are doing it in less than a year, you are 10 times smarter than me. If I can do it, anyone can.

I wish you the best of luck and we are here to help. Please reach out if we can help in any way.

There are thousands of us hoping you improve and waiting to hear your story of beating the odds.

www.stoppingkidneydisease.com

www.albutrix.com

www.kidneyhood.org

Lee

Most Common Foods

Fruit

Food	serving size (imperial)	serving size metric (g)	PRAL (Acid load) mEq/100g	protein (g)	potassium (mg)	phosphorus (mg)	sodium (mg)	Estimated ORAC
cuties, halos's, small tangerine	1.5 small	109	-3.1	0.9	181	21.8	2.2	1627
apples	1 medium	161	-1.9	0.4	145	17.7	0	3049
pears	1 medium	178	-3.9	0.6	198	18.3	1.7	1746
grapes(red and green)	25 pieces	126	0.9	0.9	241	25.2	2.5	1837
Raspberries	1 cup	123	-3	1.5	186	35.7	1.2	5065
blueberries(farm raised)	1/2 cup	75	-0.8	0.5	52.4	8.2	0.7	4669
wild blueberries	1/4 cup	28	-0.1	0.3	21	8.1	1.7	9621
blackberries	1 cup	144	-4	2	233	31.7	1.4	5905
cranberries	1 cup	100	-1.4	0.4	85	13	2	9090
bananas	1 medium	118	-8.2	1.3	422	26	1.5	795
strawberries	1 cup halves	152	-4	1	233	36.5	1.2	4302
lemons	1 medium	58	-1.4	0.6	80	9.3	1.3	1346
limes	1 medium	67	-8.2	0.5	68.3	12.1	0.5	82
apricots	1 cup, halves	155	-1.1	2.2	401	35.7	1.6	1110
nectarines	1 medium	142	-6.7	1.5	285	0	0	919
naval orange(large orange)	1 fruit	140	-4.3	1.3	232	32.2	1.4	1819
watermelon	1 wedge	286	-4.7	1.7	285	36.9	2.9	1922
cherry tomato	1 cup	149	-6.1	1.6	320	31.5	7.5	546
large tomato	1 piece	182	-7.4	1.3	431	43.7	9.1	387
peaches	1 medium	150	-4.7	1.4	353	30	0	142
canteloupe	10 balls	138	-7	1.2	368	20.7	22.1	319
honeydew melon	10 balls	138	-6.2	0.7	315	15.2	24.8	253
cherries (sweet)	1 cup with pits	138	-5.2	1.5	306	29	0	3747
pineapple	3-1/2" dia3/4" thick	84	-1.8	0.5	91.6	6.7	0.8	385
Avocados	1 cup sliced	146	-11.9	2.9	708	75.9	10.2	1922
papaya	1 cup cubes	140	-8.6	0.9	360	7	4.2	300
mango	1/2 cup	82	-2.3	0.4	128	14.1	1.6	1300
coconut meat (Fresh)	2" x2" piece	45	-1.2	1.5	160	50.8	9	20
figs(fresh not dried)	1 medium	50	-2.4	0.4	116	7	0.5	3383

Veggies

Food	serving size (imperial)	serving size metric (g)	PRAL (Acid load) mEq/100g	protein (g)	potassium (mg)	phosphorus (mg)	sodium (mg)	Estimated ORAC
white potato	1 small	170	-10.4	2.9	692	105	10.2	1058
sweet potato	1 cup cubes	133	-7.4	2.1	448	62.5	73.2	902
onions	1 medium	110	-2.2	1.2	161	31.9	4.4	913
carrots	1 large	72	-4.1	0.7	230	25.2	49.7	697
broccoli	1 stalk	151	-6	4.3	477	99.7	49.8	1510
lettuce(iceberg)	1cup, shredded	72	-1.6	0.6	102	14.4	23.7	438
spinach	1 cup	30	-3.5	0.9	167	24.1	14	1513
mustard greens	1 cup chopped	56	-3.7	1.5	198	14.7	7.2	1770
collard greens	1 cup chopped	36	-1.5	0.9	60.8	3.6	28.8	1770
kale	1 cup chopped	67	-5.6	2.2	299	37.5	1.8	1770
cilantro	1/4 cup	4	-0.4	0.1	20.8	1.9	10.2	5141
watercress	10 sprigs	25	-1.4	0.6	36.9	15	2.7	1904
arugula (rocket lettuce)	1/2 cup	10	-0.8	0.3	82.5	5.2	2.7	1904
bell peppers	1 medium	119	-4	1.2	251	30.9	4.8	821
celery	1 large and 1 medium stalk	110	-5.5	0.8	286	26.4	88	552
cucumbers	1 medium	201	-4.6	1.2	273	42.2	4	140
corn	1 medium	90	-1.6	2.9	243	80.1	13.5	728
garlic	1 clove	3	-0.1	0.2	12	4.6	0.5	5708
mushrooms	1/2 cup pieces	35	-0.8	1.1	111	30.1	1.8	691
cabbage	1 cup, shredded	70	-2	0.9	119	18.2	12.6	529
green beans	10 beans 4"long	55	-1.8	1	115	20.9	3.3	799
cauliflower	1 cup	100	-4.4	2	303	44	30	870
asparagus	1 cup or 9 spirs medium	134	-2.6	2.9	271	69.7	2.7	2252
zucchini	1 medium	196	-8.1	2.4	514	74.5	19.6	180
squash	1 cup, sliced	113	-4.7	1.4	296	42.9	2.3	396
sliced beets (canned)	1/2 cup	85	-2.3	0.75	126	14.45	165	1776
eggplant	1 cup cubes	82	-3.2	0.8	189	20.5	1.6	932

Category	Food	serving size (imperial)	Serving size metric (g)	PRAL (Acid load) mEq/100g	protein (g)	potassium (mg)	phosphorus (mg)	sodium (mg)	total fat (g)	Saturated fat (g)	total unsaturated fats (g)	Omega 3 (mg)	Omega 6 (mg)	Estimated ORAC
Veggies	artichokes (fresh)	1 medium	128	-6.4	4.2	474	115	120						6552
	artichoke hearts in water	1/2 cup	84	-2.7	2.4	240	61.3	50.4						9416
	artichoke hearts in oil	1 heart	33	-0.9	0.89	80.1	20.4	16.8						4760
	green peas	1 cup	145	0.5	7.9	354	157	7.3						260
	black eyed peas	1 cup	145	-12.5	4.3	625	76.8	5.8						4343
	jalepeno peppers	1 pepper	14	-0.5	0.2	30.1	4.3	0.1						8250
Nuts (others are too high protein)	pecans	19 halves	28	0.6	2.6	116	78.2	0						17940
	walnuts	14 halves	28	1.6	4.3	125	97.8	0.6						13541
	macadamia	10-12 kernels	28	-0.1	2.2	103	55.9	1.1						1695
Prepared foods	popcorn like smart pop	1 cup	8	0.7	1	26.3	28.6	0.6						1743
	tapioca pudding (dry)	1/2 cup	23	0	0	1.2	0.9	1.8						
	So delicious coco whip	2 tbsp	38	-0.5	0.4	38.4	8.4	13.6						
	Craisins (low sugar)	1/3 cup	40	-0.3	0	16	3.2	1.2						9090
	dried blueberries	1/4 cup	40	-1.1	1	86	14	1						4669
	dried cherries	1/4 cup	40	-2.2	1	120	0	0						3747
	dried pineapple	7 pieces	40	-0.8	0	25	0	115						385
	dried apples	1/2 cup	42	-3.5	0.4	193	16	37						6681
	raisins	1/2 cup	26	-3.1	0.8	195	26.3	2.9						3406
	dried figs	3.5 figs	28	-3.9	0.9	190	18.8	2.8						3383
	prunes	3 pitted	28	-3.8	0.6	205	19.3	0.6						8059
	dried mangos	4 pieces	40	-1.3	0.98	112	20	65						1300
	sun dried tomatos	1/2 cup	28	-16.3	4	960	99.7	587						423
	dried coconut	4.5 tbsp	28	-0.9	1.9	152	57.7	10.4						90
Drinks	black tea	1 cup	237	-1.9	0	87.7	2.4	7.1						1128
	green tea	12 fl oz	340	0	0	0	0	5						520
	chai tea	12 fl oz	340	0.7	0	0	0	80						313
	Black coffee	6 fl oz	179	-1.1	0.2			7.2						2780
	rice milk	1 cup	244	-0.4	0.67	65	94	94	2					30
	oat milk	1 cup	240	-1.8	2	95		105						1708
	almond milk	8 fl oz or 1 cup	240	-8.2	1.51	35	46	105						1708
	coconut milk beverage	1 cup	240	-4.5		631	240	36						90
	soy creamer	1 container, individual	15	-0.2		28.6								
	soy milk beverage	1 cup	243	0.2	7.95	287	126	124						5409
	hemp milk beverage	1 cup	240	5.5	3	170	451	134						9800
	cashew milk beverage	1 cup	240	-2.1	1	25	134	160			not found			1948
	100% juice cranberry juice	1 cup	253	-3	1	195	32.9	5.1			not found			865
	Concord grape juice	1 cup	253	-4.8	0.9	263	35.4	12.7						2389
	apple juice	1 cup	248	-5.1	0.2	251	17.4	9.9						414
	pear nectar	1 cup	250	-0.6	0.3	32.5	7.5	10						704
	pineapple juice	1 cup	250	-6.8	0.9	325	20	5						568
	orange juice	1 cup	249	-8.2	1.7	458	42.3	10						726
	hibiscus tea homemade	1 cup	236	-1.3	0	47	2	9						6990

Oils

Food	Serving size Imperial	Metric (g)	Calories					total fat (g)	Saturated fat (g)	total unsaturated fats (g)	Omega 3 (mg)	Omega 6 (mg)	
Canola oil	1 tbsp	14	119					13.5	1	11.9	1031	2532	
vegetable oil	1 tbsp	14	119					13.5	3.3	9.6	28.2	1160	
avocado oil	1 tbsp	14	124					14	1.6	11.8	134	1754	
smart balance oil	1 tbsp	14	120					14	1	12.5	990	0	
olive oil	1 tbsp	14	119					13.5	1.9	11.2	103	1318	
grapeseed oil	1 tbsp	14	119					13.5	1.3	11.6	13.5	9395	
flaxseed oil	1 tbsp	14	119					13.5	1.3	11.6	7196	1715	
coconut oil	1 tbsp	14	116					13.5	11.7	1	trace	243	
walnut oil	1 tbsp	14	119					13.5	1.2	11.6	1404	7141	
sesame oil	1 tbsp	14	119					13.6	1.9	11	40.5	5576	
Safflower oil	1 tbsp	14	119					13.5	0.8	12	trace	10073	
Sunflower oil	1 tbsp	14	119					13.5	1.2	11.6	5	3905	
Corn oil	1 tbsp	14	100					13.5	1.7	11.1	157	7224	
Butter	1 tbsp	14	119					11.4	7.2	10.1	44.1	382	
palm oil	1 tbsp	14	116					13.5	11	1.7	trace	216	

INDEX

RECIPES BY PREPARATION TIME

Preparation time under 5 minutes

Preparation time under 10 minutes

Preparation time under 15 minutes

Preparation time under 20 minutes

Preparation time under 25 minutes

RECIPES BY COOK TIME

Cook time under 5 minutes

Charred Romaine with Caesar Dressing, 68

Fresh Fruit with Vanilla Syrup, 93

Marinated Carrot Salad, 78

Matcha Latte, 98

Mexican Street Corn Salad, 84

Thai Pineapple Salad with Carrot Cashew Dressing, 61

Vegetable Masala, 62

Cook time under 10 minutes

Blåbärssoppa, 39

Blackberry Iced Tea, 97

Macadamia Freezer Fudge, 88

Omelet Huevo Ranchero, 44

Shakshuka, 46

Stewed Cinnamon Apples, 43

Cook time under 15 minutes

Coconut Macaroons, 90

Hibiscus Tea, 96

Raspberry Fool, 91

Smoky Collard Greens, 54

Cook time under 20 minutes

Beet Salad with Candied or Spiced Pecans, 51

Creamy Breakfast Polenta with Stewed Blackberries, 41

Ginger-Garlic Vegetable Ramen Bowls, 71

Italian Pesto Zucchini Noodles, 82

Jackfruit "Carnitas" Tacos, 69

Jackfruit Crab Cakes, 79

Pineapple and Vegetable Kebabs, 67

Pineapple with Rum Sauce, 92

Tortilla Soup, 70

Vegetable Fajitas, 83

Cook time under 25 minutes

Baked Sweet Potato with Side Salad, 57

Pumpkin Chili, 56

Tostada Salad, 55

Cook time under 30 minutes

Corn and Chile Soup with Smoky Collard Greens, 53

Gumbo Z'Herbes, 63

Mushroom Bourguignon, 74

Pears in Wine Sauce, 89

Pepper Salad, 76

Portobello Steaks, 65

Cook time under 35 minutes

Pumpkin Soup with "Chorizo" Mushrooms & Corn, 59

Cook time under 40 minutes

Fruit Ice Cream, 85

RECIPES BY PRICE

Meals for up to $1.00

Blackberry Iced Tea, 97

Blackberry Sangria Granita, 94

Charred Romaine with Caesar Dressing, 68

Cherry Lemonade, 95

Coconut Macaroons, 90

Fruit Ice Cream, 86

Hibiscus Tea, 96

Louisiana Remoulade, 80

Macadamia Freezer Fudge, 88

Matcha Latte, 98

Mexican Street Corn Salad, 84

Pineapple with Rum Sauce, 92

Raspberry Fool, 91

Smoky Collard Greens, 54

Meals for up to $2.00

Baked Sweet Potato with Side Salad, 58

Creamy Breakfast Polenta with Stewed Blackberries, 42

Fresh Fruit with Vanilla Syrup, 93

Fruit and Trail Mix, 99

Marinated Carrot Salad, 78

Pecan and Fruit Bowls, 48

Pineapple and Vegetable Kebabs, 67

Stewed Cinnamon Apples, 43

Tortilla Soup, 70

Tostada Salad, 55

Vinegar Slaw, 81

Watermelon-Blueberry Sorbet, 87

Meals for up to $3.00

Basic Fruit Smoothie, 50

Corn and Chile Soup, 53

Green Pineapple Smoothie, 49

Gumbo Z'Herbes, 64

Italian Pesto Zucchini Noodles, 82

Main Dish Salad, 73

No-Sodium Umami Sauce, 72

Omelet Huevo Ranchero, 45

Pears in Wine Sauce, 89

Pepper Salad, 76

Portobello Steaks with Twice-Cooked Mashed Potatoes (or cauliflower) and Balsamic Arugula Salad, 66

Pumpkin Chili, 56

Pumpkin Soup with "Chorizo" Mushrooms & Corn, 60

Shakshuka, 46

Vegetable Fajitas, 83

Vegetable Masala, 62

Meals for up to $4.00

Jackfruit "Carnitas" Tacos, 69

Jackfruit Crab Cakes, 79

Mushroom Bourguignon, 74

Thai Pineapple Salad with Carrot Cashew Dressing, 61

Watermelon Gazpacho, 77

REFERENCES

1. Lemos CF, Rodrigues MP, Veiga JRP. Family income is associated with quality of life in patients with chronic kidney disease in the pre-dialysis phase: a cross sectional study. *Health and quality of life outcomes.* 2015;13(1):202.

2. Kalantar-Zadeh K, Kilpatrick RD, Kuwae N, et al. Revisiting mortality predictability of serum albumin in the dialysis population: time dependency, longitudinal changes and population-attributable fraction. *Nephrology Dialysis Transplantation.* 2005;20(9):1880-1888.

3. Pupim LB, Caglar K, Hakim RM, Shyr Y, Ikizler TA. Uremic malnutrition is a predictor of death independent of inflammatory status. *Kidney International.* 2004;66(5):2054-2060.

4. Watford M. Glutamine and glutamate: Nonessential or essential amino acids? *Animal Nutrition.* 2015;1(3):119-122.

5. Bonanni A, Mannucci I, Verzola D, et al. Protein-energy wasting and mortality in chronic kidney disease. *International journal of environmental research and public health.* 2011;8(5):1631-1654.

6. Castiglia PT. Protein-energy malnutrition (kwashiorkor and marasmus). *Journal of Pediatric Health Care.* 1996;10(1):28-30.

7. Olsen NS, Bassett JW. Blood levels of urea nitrogen, phenol, guanidine and creatinine in uremia. *The American journal of medicine.* 1951;10(1):52-59.

8. Kovesdy CP, Kopple JD, Kalantar-Zadeh K. Management of protein-energy wasting in non-dialysis-dependent chronic kidney disease: reconciling low protein intake with nutritional therapy–. *The American Journal of Clinical Nutrition.* 2013;97(6):1163-1177.

9. Kalender B. Malnutrition in chronic kidney disease and relationship to quality of life. *Handbook of Disease Burdens and Quality of Life Measures.* 2010:3159-3170.

10. Prior RL. Oxygen radical absorbance capacity (ORAC): New horizons in relating dietary antioxidants/bioactives and health benefits. *Journal of Functional Foods.* 2015;18:797-810.

11. Oberg BP, McMenamin E, Lucas F, et al. Increased prevalence of oxidant stress and inflammation in patients with moderate to severe chronic kidney disease. *Kidney International.* 2004;65(3):1009-1016.

The first book by Lee Hull and Kidneyhood.org is *Stopping Kidney Disease*

Stopping Kidney Disease is the most comprehensive guide to understanding how your kidneys work and how to make your remaining kidney function last as long as possible. The book includes over 500 pages with hundreds of medical studies to document each part of the diet and treatment plan.

As a patient trying to cure an incurable kidney disease, Lee Hull was not allowed access to a potential life-saving treatment when other patients had access to the same medicine/supplement. He found that outcomes for a kidney patient vary widely dependent on the country and even state you live in. Lee was able to put his kidney disease in remission by using the treatment plan and diet in *Stopping Kidney Disease*. He decided to write this book and share what he has learned after living successfully with incurable kidney disease for over twenty years.

Lee believes everyone deserves the right to try and stop an incurable disease regardless of where you live or your net worth. The project Kidneyhood.org is trying to provide education and innovation to help kidney patients worldwide slow the progression of their disease.

For more information and to sign up for free updates to *Stopping Kidney Disease*, kidney friendly recipes, patient success stories and research for kidney patients, visit:

stoppingkidneydisease.com

The Kidneyhood.org books can be found on Amazon as well as all other online retailers.